Engagement and Therapeutic Communication in Mental Health Nursing

Transforming Nursing Practice series

Transforming Nursing Practice is the first series of books designed to help students meet the requirements of the NMC Standards and Essential Skills Clusters for degree programmes. Each book addresses a core topic, and together they cover the generic knowledge required for all fields of practice.

Core knowledge titles:

Series editor: Professor Shirley Bach, Head of the School of Health Sciences at the University of Brighton

Acute and Critical Care in Adult Nursing	ISBN 978 0 85725 842 7
Becoming a Registered Nurse: Making the Transition to Practice	ISBN 978 0 85725 931 8
Caring for Older People in Nursing	ISBN 978 1 44626 763 9
Communication and Interpersonal Skills in Nursing (2nd edn)	ISBN 978 0 85725 449 8
Contexts of Contemporary Nursing (2nd edn)	ISBN 978 1 84445 374 0
Dementia Care in Nursing	ISBN 978 0 85725 873 1
Getting into Nursing	ISBN 978 0 85725 895 3
Health Promotion and Public Health for Nursing Students (2nd edn)	ISBN 978 1 44627 503 0
Introduction to Medicines Management in Nursing	ISBN 978 1 84445 845 5
Law and Professional Issues in Nursing (3rd edn)	ISBN 978 1 44626 858 2
Leadership, Management and Team Working in Nursing	ISBN 978 0 85725 453 5
Learning Skills for Nursing Students	ISBN 978 1 84445 376 4
Medicines Management in Adult Nursing	ISBN 978 1 84445 842 4
Medicines Management in Children's Nursing	ISBN 978 1 84445 470 9
Nursing Adults with Long Term Conditions	ISBN 978 0 85725 441 2
Nursing and Collaborative Practice (2nd edn)	ISBN 978 1 84445 373 3
Nursing and Mental Health Care	ISBN 978 1 84445 467 9
Passing Calculations Tests for Nursing Students (2nd edn)	ISBN 978 1 44625 642 8
Patient and Carer Participation in Nursing	ISBN 978 0 85725 307 1
Patient Assessment and Care Planning in Nursing	ISBN 978 0 85725 858 8
Patient Safety and Managing Risk in Nursing	ISBN 978 1 44626 688 5
Psychology and Sociology in Nursing	ISBN 978 0 85725 836 6
Safeguarding Adults in Nursing Practice	ISBN 978 1 44625 638 1
Successful Practice Learning for Nursing Students (2nd edn)	ISBN 978 0 85725 315 6
Using Health Policy in Nursing	ISBN 978 1 44625 646 6
What is Nursing? Exploring Theory and Practice (3rd edn)	ISBN 978 0 85725 975 2

Personal and professional learning skills titles:

Series editors: Dr Mooi Standing, Independent Academic Consultant (UK and International) & Accredited NMC Reviewer, and Professor Shirley Bach, Head of the School of Health Sciences at the University of Brighton

Clinical Judgement and Decision Making in Nursing (2nd edn)	ISBN 978 1 44628 281 6
Critical Thinking and Writing for Nursing Students (2nd edn)	ISBN 978 1 44625 644 2
Evidence-based Practice in Nursing (2nd edn)	ISBN 978 1 44627 090 5
Information Skills for Nursing Students	ISBN 978 1 84445 381 8
Reflective Practice in Nursing (2nd edn)	ISBN 978 1 44627 085 1
Succeeding in Essays, Exams & OSCEs for Nursing Students	ISBN 978 0 85725 827 4
Succeeding in Research Project Plans and Literature Reviews for Nursing Students	ISBN 978 0 85725 264 7
Successful Professional Portfolios for Nursing Students	ISBN 978 0 85725 457 3
Understanding Research for Nursing Students (2nd edn)	ISBN 978 1 44626 761 5

Mental health nursing titles:

Series editors: Sandra Walker, Senior Teaching Fellow in Mental Health in the Faculty of Health Sciences, University of Southampton, and Professor Shirley Bach, Head of the School of Health Sciences at the University of Brighton

Assessment and Decision Making in Mental Health Nursing	ISBN 978 1 44626 820 9
Engagement and Therapeutic Communication in Mental Health Nursing	ISBN 978 1 44627 480 4
Medicines Management in Mental Health Nursing	ISBN 978 0 85725 049 0
Mental Health Law in Nursing	ISBN 978 0 85725 761 1

You can find more information on each of these titles and our other learning resources at www.sagepub.co.uk. Many of these titles are also available in various e-book formats; please visit our website for more information.

Engagement and Therapeutic Communication in Mental Health Nursing

Edited by
Sandra Walker

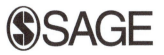 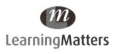

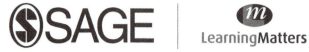

Learning Matters
An imprint of SAGE Publications Ltd
1 Oliver's Yard
55 City Road
London EC1Y 1SP

SAGE Publications Inc.
2455 Teller Road
Thousand Oaks, California 91320

SAGE Publications India Pvt Ltd
B 1/I 1 Mohan Cooperative Industrial Area
Mathura Road
New Delhi 110 044

SAGE Publications Asia-Pacific Pte Ltd
3 Church Street
#10–04 Samsung Hub
Singapore 049483

Editor: Alex Clabburn
Development editor: Caroline Sheldrick
Production controller: Chris Marke
Project management: Diana Chambers
Marketing manager: Tamara Navaratnam
Cover design: Wendy Scott
Typeset by: Kelly Winter
Copy editor: Sue Edwards
Printed and bound by CPI Group (UK) Ltd,
Croydon, CR0 4YY

Library of Congress Control Number: 2014932989

British Library Cataloguing in Publication Data
A catalogue record for this book is available from
the British Library

ISBN: 978 1 4462 7480 4

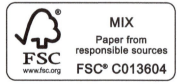

MIX
Paper from
responsible sources
FSC® C013604
www.fsc.org

Contents

Foreword

One thing that can never be overlooked in mental healthcare is the complexity of human beings. Unfailingly individual, we all operate from a comprehensive array of cultural backgrounds and beliefs; various levels of knowledge and understanding; differing likes and dislikes; diverse life experiences and multiple behaviours. Learning to navigate these differences and managing to connect with others despite them, is one of the hardest tasks ahead of us in our quest for high quality care for those in mental distress. Research has consistently shown that it is the human relationships we develop that have the biggest impact on recovery in mental healthcare; successful engagement and therapeutic communication are essential in order to help people find their way out of the maze of problems that may have beset them.

This book offers many practical suggestions as to how to ensure we successfully engage with those in our care, underpinned by a broad base of theory and evidence. The principles of person-centred recovery, validation, respect and dignity are themes that are interwoven throughout the chapters. The book provides practical exercises that will help the reader to develop a stronger sense of self both as a person and a professional while at the same time learning to put themselves in the shoes of the person they are caring for and always remembering that it is their values, not ours, that must direct our action.

There are two outstanding themes, however, that bear further consideration as you embark on reading this text. The *importance of self-awareness* is a recurring theme throughout the chapters. It is essential that we are aware of our own cultural background, our own values, beliefs and attitudes, our non-verbal body language, our limitations and when we need to ask for help. The importance of supervision and reflective practice support this and are repeatedly highlighted as hallmarks of best practice. Additionally, *curiosity* is another, often reoccurring, theme. It is the way to ensure we are not hijacked by our own standpoint. To ask gentle probing questions of the position of the person in distress, to maintain a respectful curiosity in the face of behaviour we find difficult to understand, is key in helping us to work collaboratively with people to help them recover. The importance of these two themes cannot be underestimated.

If you are a student nurse, a newly qualified nurse or even a nurse of some years' standing looking for tips to update your portfolio of skills, this book will stand you in good stead for practice. It can be read as a whole but can also be dipped into section by section as you come across situations in practice, perhaps, that warrant further exploration of that particular subject. Engaging with this book will help you to become a more effective practitioner of the art of mental health nursing, enhancing your ability to connect with people of diverse backgrounds and needs.

Sandra Walker
April 2014

Acknowledgements

The authors and publisher wish to thank the following for permission to reproduce copyright material.

Open University Press for the nursing qualities displayed in Figure 1.1, from Megan Ellis and Crispen Day (2013) The therapeutic relationship: engaging clients in their care and treatment, Chapter 12 in Norman, IJ and Ryrie, I (eds) *The Art and Science of Mental Health Nursing: Principles and practice*, pp172 and 174.

David A Richards and Mark Whyte (2011) for Figures 4.1 and 4.2, Funnelling, reproduced with kind permission from *Reach Out: National Programme Student Materials to Support the Delivery of Training for Psychological Wellbeing Practitioners Delivering Low Intensity Interventions* (3rd Edition). London: Rethink.

About the authors

Peter Bullard is the Accredited Psychological Wellbeing Practitioner (PWP) Quality Lead for the Isle of Wight Primary Care Mental Health service. He works with individuals suffering from anxiety and depression, and delivers low-intensity CBT interventions through different modalities. He graduated from Southampton University in 2010 and has worked on the course as a clinical educator since that year. He has an MSc in Transcultural Mental Health and Psychological Therapies. Before working in mental health services he had a background in physical fitness, completing his degree in Health and Fitness management, and working as an instructor and trainer in many different healthcare settings. He strongly believes in the value of combining therapeutic approaches with the application of improving well-being for individuals experiencing mental health problems.

Simon Grist is a Lecturer in Mental Health and Programme Lead for the Improving Access to Psychological Therapies Psychological Wellbeing Practitioner programme at the University of Southampton. A qualified mental health nurse and CBT therapist, prior to working at the university he was a CMHT manager, working extensively in crisis and home treatment teams and in substance misuse services.

Yvonne Middlewick has been a mental health lecturer within the University of Southampton for six years. A dual registered nurse, RGN and RMN, she has had a varied career working with people of different ages. She started her career in a gynaecology and breast surgery unit, where she cared for people with complex psychological as well as physiological needs, rekindling her interest in mental health. As a result, she completed a post-qualifying mental health course at Bournemouth University, and later worked with older adults in a mental health setting before returning to an adult nursing environment to work with older people. Experience from both settings has helped Yvonne to holistically care for older people with complex needs.

Dorothy Neal is a pseudonym used, at her request, to protect the identity of the service user who co-wrote her chapter. She has a long history of mental health problems as well as a full and active family life plus a love of dancing.

Julia Pelle is a Senior Lecturer in Mental Health Nursing at Kingston University and St George's University London. She currently teaches on culture, ethnicity and diversity in mental health and social care to pre- and post-registration students. Julia maintains a research interest in family carers from Black and Ethnic Minority communities who care for relatives with an enduring mental health problem. She also worked as a Senior Nurse in an acute inpatient mental health setting before moving into health and social care education.

Wendy Turton (RMN, MSc, BABCP Accred. Cognitive Therapist) is currently a Lecturer in Mental Health within the Faculty of Health Sciences at the University of Southampton and the Senior Psychological Therapist with a Mental Health Recovery Team in Portsmouth. Wendy trained in Leicestershire on an integrated Mental Health and Learning Disability nursing programme, choosing to focus her career on mental health, and in recent years on severe and enduring mental health problems, in particular the experience of psychosis. In 2004 Wendy set up the Psychosocial Interventions for Psychosis Service (PSIPS) within South East Hampshire, which she led for nine years. During this time Wendy was involved in clinical research, exploring the efficacy of *Person-based Cognitive Therapy for Distressing Psychosis* (Chadwick, 2006) and co-authored two award-winning short books on the experience of living with psychosis with MH service users; her ongoing research continues to focus on the lived experience of psychosis. Wendy also works with the CBT Programme Team at the University of Southampton.

Sandra Walker is a Senior Teaching Fellow in Mental Health at Southampton University, where she is also a doctorate student researching the patient experience of the mental health assessment in the Emergency Department. She is a Qualified Mental Health Nurse with a wide range of clinical experience spanning more than 20 years. In addition to her university work, she is a professional musician and does voluntary work for various mental health organisations, including being the coordinator for the Hampshire Human Library – an international initiative aimed at reducing stigma through interaction and education of the public. She is the creative director of The Sanity Company, which publishes books aimed at helping children and young people develop good mental health and problem-solving skills.

Janine Ward is an accredited Psychological Wellbeing Practitioner (PWP) and Mental Health Practitioner by background and has worked within forensic mental health, learning difficulties, community mental health and substance abuse teams. Janine currently leads the Southampton Improving Access to Psychological Therapies Low Intensity and Assessment Team and provides some clinical leadership across her employing Trust. She is seconded as a PWP educator at the University of Southampton and has worked within the Health Sciences Faculty for the last three years. Janine is currently studying for her PhD at Southampton.

Andy Williams joined the Royal Navy at 18 and served for 22 years, during which time he trained as a Registered General Nurse and later a Registered Mental Nurse. Andy is a Master of Arts in Mental Health and a Bachelor of Nursing with Education in order to register for the education of nurses. On leaving the service, Andy secured a senior lecturer post with the MOD before accepting a post at Southampton University.

Andy's teaching interests are in interpersonal and communication skills, bereavement and loss, post-traumatic stress disorder, spirituality, adult mental health, particularly around anxiety and depression, suicide and self-harm. He is involved in nurse education in pre- and post-qualifying programmes and IAPT education.

Introduction

About this book

This book is written primarily for student nurses currently undertaking their qualifications. It will also be useful for junior nurses who are just beginning their careers and would be a useful refresher for anyone who cares for people in mental distress on a regular basis.

Why *Engagement and Therapeutic Communication?*

Building a good rapport with service users is essential to good mental healthcare. This book explores simple techniques to facilitate this and encourages readers to reflect on their own communication styles and become more aware of how their communications affect others. There is a lot of theoretical material available on communication and engagement; however, this book aims to provide a more active and engaging experience and case studies that will allow the reader to practise some of the techniques shared in the context of recovery, which is a core underpinning of this book. The NMC *Standards for Pre-registration Nursing Education* (2010a) demand that, for mental health nurses, 'therapeutic use of self' is essential in providing high-quality care (Competencies for entry to the register: Mental health nursing, Domain 2: Communication and interpersonal skills, Field standard for competence). The skills required to do this are challenging, especially as the environment of healthcare is becoming increasingly pressured.

This book introduces the basic elements of communication in mental health nursing and provides readers with material to help them develop excellent engagement skills and begin to discover what 'therapeutic use of self' means to them. The NMC *Standards for Pre-registration Nursing Education* (2010a), to which all programmes must comply by 2014, require that students must have acquired by the end of their training 'communication and interpersonal skills' as a core element in their nursing practice. The new standards contain more detailed requirements for communication and interpersonal skills than the previous standards, and there are specific requirements for mental health nurses. This book covers content outlined in these requirements for mental health nurses specifically, and is an excellent tool in assisting the development of these skills.

Book structure

In Chapter 1 we are introduced to communication in mental health, including communication styles and what advanced communication is. It starts out to draw a comparison that allows the reader to begin to distinguish between straightforward communication and therapeutic communication. The elements of therapeutic communication are explored along with considerations as to how therapeutic communications can be improved by developing self-awareness through supervision. There is a first look at how best to communicate with people in distress, those who have experienced abuse or traumatic events and people in psychotic states.

Chapter 2 looks at the issue of engagement. The main concepts of therapeutic engagement are described and why good engagement skills are a key element of the role of the mental health nurse. This chapter articulates the interpersonal dynamics of the process of engagement and the importance of increased self-awareness when initiating therapeutic relationships with service users. The importance of a person-centred approach to care is examined along with how this underpins effective engagement skills. This allows for application of a developed understanding of therapeutic engagement in your practice.

In Chapter 3, building rapport, including therapeutic use of self, is the focus. The importance of the therapeutic alliance is stressed in helping service users fully understand their techniques, rationales and values in helping them reach their goals. The need for an intervention to be adaptable to the service user's needs without sacrificing professional standards is an issue considered here, as well as the importance of collaboration with the service user having a say in all decisions. Efforts to enhance the relationship should be considered throughout the intervention or risk losing the power to make change. It is emphasised that the mental health nurse should try to understand the service user from his or her unique perspective, even if the nurse feels the service user needs to be challenged. As part of this the importance of avoiding criticism, blame and rejection and instead maintaining a curious stance are emphasised.

Chapter 4 looks at the practical issue of questioning techniques, including downward arrowing or funnelling. Here a range of questioning styles to communicate with service users are considered in order to reflect, paraphrase, clarify and summarise in order to allow the reader to learn ways to gather appropriate and relevant information in a timely manner.

What helps when communication becomes difficult is the focus of Chapter 5, including cognitive impairment and psychosis. There is an exploration of the factors that can affect communication and make it more difficult in mental health nursing. We begin to recognise the effects that being cognitively impaired can have on communication. This chapter also encourages reflection on your own assumptions, values and beliefs, and their impact on how you communicate with others. Some strategies are described that may help to break down some of the barriers to communication.

Chapter 6 considers issues related to cross-cultural communication. It defines and identifies barriers to cross-cultural communication in mental healthcare. This chapter starts with a general introduction to cross-cultural communication in mental healthcare, followed by a review of the barrier to the delivery of cross-cultural communication. An overview of the effective communication strategies used in mental health practice is discussed and the significant role of the mental health nurse in implementing these strategies underpins the wider debate around cross-cultural communication.

Chapter 7 continues this cross-cultural journey but from the perspective of the carer as partner in care. This chapter explores how carers, usually family members or friends, become important in supporting the delivery of health and social care to different client groups. Some time is spent reviewing the meaning of 'carer', and how carers work in partnership with mental health nurses is the theme throughout the chapter. A definition of 'partnership' is provided in the context of mental health and social care practice. The partnership approach to involving carers in care for others requires that the nurse assesses the health and social care needs of carers, who may experience the burden of caring over time as well as trying to adjust to their roles as carers. Ensuring that there are equal opportunities to receive support from health and social care services indicates that nurses need to focus on carer groups that may not be reached due to stigma, social exclusion and discrimination, for example young carers, carers who are economically disadvantaged, carers from black and ethnic minority communities, and carers from lesbian, gay, bisexual and transgendered communities.

In the last chapter, the service user perspective is the focus of attention – why it's important to get it right! This chapter is slightly unusual in format in that it is presented primarily as one case study, comprising an interview carried out with a service user, following several years of care in a variety of clinical settings. Into this interview are interspersed activities, reflections and alternative case studies to help you to think more broadly around the issues raised within the interview itself, including how the clinicians' behaviour impacts on care delivery, and the ethical issues arising from a given clinical situation. It also encourages reflection on your own values and judgements in interacting with service users in day-to-day care in the hope that, by the end of the chapter and indeed this book, you will have an increased understanding of the importance of validation and maintaining dignity in clinical care.

Requirements for the NMC *Standards for Pre-registration Nursing Education* and the Essential Skills Clusters

The Nursing and Midwifery Council (NMC) has established standards of competence to be met by applicants to different parts of the register, and these are the standards it considers necessary for safe and effective practice. In addition to the competencies, the NMC has set out specific skills that nursing students must be able to perform at various points of an education programme. These are known as Essential Skills Clusters (ESCs). This book is structured so that it will help you to understand and meet the competencies and ESCs required for entry to the NMC register. The relevant competencies and ESCs are presented at the start of each chapter so that you can clearly see which ones the chapter addresses. There are *generic standards* that all nursing students irrespective of their field must achieve, and *field-specific standards* relating to each field of nursing, that is, mental health, children's, learning disability and adult nursing. Most chapters have generic standards, and occasionally field-specific standards are listed.

This book includes the latest standards for 2010 onwards, taken from *Standards for Pre-registration Nursing Education* (NMC, 2010a).

Learning features

Throughout the book you will find activities in the text that will help you to make sense of, and learn about, the material being presented by the authors.

Some activities ask you to reflect on aspects of practice, or your experience of it, or the people or situations you encounter. *Reflection* is an essential skill in nursing, and it helps you to understand the world around you and often to identify how things might be improved. Other activities will help you develop key skills such as your ability to *think critically* about a topic in order to challenge received wisdom, or your ability to *research a topic and find appropriate information and evidence*, and to be able to make decisions using that evidence in situations that are often difficult and time-pressured. Finally, communication and working as part of a team are core to all nursing practice, and some activities will ask you to think about your *communication skills* to help develop these skills.

All the activities require you to take a break from reading the text, think through the issues presented and carry out some independent study, possibly using the internet. Where appropriate, there are sample answers presented at the end of each chapter, and these will help you to understand more fully your own reflections and independent study. Remember, academic study will always require independent work; attending lectures will never be enough to be successful on your programme, and these activities will help to deepen your knowledge and understanding of the issues under scrutiny and give you practice at working on your own.

You might want to think about completing these activities as part of your personal development plan (PDP) or portfolio. After completing the activity, write it up in your PDP or portfolio in a section devoted to that particular skill, then look back over time to see how far you have developed. You can also do more of the activities for a key skill that you have identified a weakness in, which will help build your skill and confidence in this area.

It is the aim of this book to use an interactive style with realistic scenarios, to be a book that explains how, as well as why, while taking account of the complexity of modern healthcare, thereby providing the reader with practical tools to add to his or her toolbox of communication skills.

Chapter 1
Therapeutic communication in mental health nursing

Andy Williams

NMC Standards for Pre-registration Nursing Education

This chapter will address the following competencies:

Domain 2: Communication and interpersonal skills

> **Mental health nurses** must practise in a way that focuses on the therapeutic use of self. They must draw on a range of methods of engaging with people of all ages experiencing mental health problems, and those important to them, to develop and maintain therapeutic relationships. They must work alongside people, using a range of interpersonal approaches and skills to help them explore and make sense of their experiences in a way that promotes recovery.

1. All nurses must build partnerships and therapeutic relationships through safe, effective and non-discriminatory communication. They must take account of individual differences, capabilities and needs.

1.1 **Mental health nurses** must use skills of relationship-building and communication to engage with and support people distressed by hearing voices, experiencing distressing thoughts or experiencing other perceptual problems.

4. All nurses must recognise when people are anxious or in distress and respond effectively, using therapeutic principles, to promote their wellbeing, manage personal safety and resolve conflict. They must use effective communication strategies and negotiation techniques to achieve best outcomes, respecting the dignity and human rights of all concerned. They must know when to consult a third party and how to make referrals for advocacy, mediation or arbitration.

4.1 **Mental health nurses** must be sensitive to, and take account of, the impact of abuse and trauma on people's wellbeing and the development of mental health problems. They must use interpersonal skills and make interventions that help people disclose and discuss their experiences as part of their recovery.

5. All nurses must use therapeutic principles to engage, maintain and, where appropriate, disengage from professional caring relationships, and must always respect professional boundaries.

5.1 **Mental health nurses** must use their personal qualities, experiences and interpersonal skills to develop and maintain therapeutic, recovery-focused relationships with people and therapeutic groups. They must be aware of their own mental health, and

continued . . .

know when to share aspects of their own life to inspire hope while maintaining professional boundaries.

Domain 3: Nursing practice and decision-making

7.1 **Mental health nurses** must provide support and therapeutic interventions for people experiencing critical and acute mental health problems. They must recognise the health and social factors that can contribute to crisis and relapse and use skills in early intervention, crisis resolution and relapse management in a way that ensures safety and security and promotes recovery.

8. All nurses must provide educational support, facilitation skills and therapeutic nursing interventions to optimise health and wellbeing. They must promote self-care and management whenever possible, helping people to make choices about their healthcare needs, involving families and carers where appropriate, to maximise their ability to care for themselves.

NMC Essential Skills Clusters

This chapter will address the following ESCs:

Cluster: Care, compassion and communication

1. As partners in the care process, people can trust a newly registered graduate nurse to provide collaborative care based on the highest standards, knowledge and competence.

By the first progression point:

4. Shows respect for others.
5. Is able to engage with people and build caring professional relationships.

By the second progression point:

6. Forms appropriate and constructive professional relationships with families and their carers.

By entry to the register:

11. Acts as a role model in developing trusting relationships, within professional boundaries.
12. Recognises and acts to overcome barriers in developing effective relationships with service users and carers.

13. People can trust the newly registered graduate nurse to respect them as individuals and strive to help them the preserve their dignity at all times.

By the first progression point:

3. Uses ways to maximise communication where hearing, vision or speech is compromised.

continued . . .

5. People can trust the newly registered graduate nurse to engage with them in a warm, sensitive and compassionate way.

6. People can trust the newly registered graduate nurse to engage therapeutically and actively listen to their needs and concerns, responding using skills that are helpful, providing information that is clear, accurate, meaningful and free from jargon.

By entry to the register:

7. Consistently shows ability to communicate safely and effectively with people providing guidance for others.

8. Communicates effectively and sensitively in different settings, using a range of methods and skills.

9. Provides accurate and comprehensive written and verbal reports based on best available evidence.

10. Acts autonomously to reduce and challenge barriers to effective communication and understanding.

11. Is proactive and creative in enhancing communication and understanding.

12. Uses the skills of active listening, questioning, paraphrasing and reflection to support a therapeutic intervention.

Chapter aims

By the end of this chapter you should be able to:

- distinguish between communication and therapeutic communication;
- describe determinants of therapeutic communication;
- describe how you can improve therapeutic communications by developing self-awareness through supervision;
- communicate with people in distress, who have experienced abuse or traumatic events;
- know how to communicate with people in psychotic states.

Introduction

Welcome to the world of mental health nursing. You are entering a healthcare field where you will be caring for vulnerable people who experience mental dysfunction, disease or illness. The nature of the dysfunction may be acute or long term, severe or less severe or an acute exacerbation of a long-term illness. Your patients will be in a range of settings, which will include forensic units, inpatient wards, community settings or their own homes. You will care for patients across the age span – young people, elderly and adult. Your patients will present with a range of human emotions, some of which will be exaggerated; for example, patients with bipolar disorder may at times be very elated in mood and extreme in aggressive behaviours. Some patients will express bizarre thoughts and behave in inappropriate, antisocial or unusual and sometimes disturbing ways. Some will have experienced particularly traumatic life events, or will have been the victims of abuse, and will be disturbed by painful images and memories.

This may all sound rather daunting; however, in preparing to become a mental health nurse, you have entered a programme of nurse education that will equip you with the essential knowledge and skills in order to be effective in your role. The heart of mental health nursing is in the relationship identified by Hildegard Peplau (1952), a leading light in the development of theory and practice focused on the interpersonal nature of nursing in mental healthcare. In order to achieve this, it is essential to develop the background knowledge and skills in communication, and a range of interpersonal skills in order to engage effectively to initiate and sustain therapeutic relationships with patients and their carers.

You will be working as part of nursing and interdisciplinary teams and therefore will need to develop skills of effective communication with colleagues in order to contribute to the overall care your patient is receiving. Effective communication between individuals and teams responsible for patient care can only enhance the care that the patient will receive. Since Peplau's early works, there have been extensive writings in the area of communication through to interpersonal skills, counselling and therapies that interrelate covering an array of skills and approaches. The recent publication of the '6Cs' by the Chief Nurse, Jane Cummings (2012), complements and supports the notion of an interpersonal skills model of nursing. The behaviours and activities of nurses in delivering care with an underpinning of therapeutic intervention are an absolute must. This chapter can only begin to scratch the surface and will focus on the development of the interpersonal relationship of nursing, seeking to address the NMC (2010a) competences and Essential Skills Clusters related to this.

The basics of communication

Before we look at therapeutic communication and therapeutic relationships, it is important to return to basics and explore the fundamentals of communication theory.

'No man is an island' – the classic words of John Donne iterate the fact that we are not meant to live alone and, while one reads of the odd recluse, generally we have others around us. As human beings, we live and work in social groupings and, in order to maintain harmony, it is important that we 'get along with' and 'fit in'. Through developments over the last couple of centuries and into the very technological world of today, there has been huge growth in the variety and means by which we can communicate as our communication has extended much more globally. From the early nineteenth century, inventions such as the radio, television, telephones and mobile phones have enabled us to reach further afield. The ability to send and receive text messages, satellite communication, computers and WiFi, and a host of networking media such as Facebook and Twitter and, of course, email, have further extended this. The science of communication and the means or channels through which we communicate have grown immensely.

Despite all the technology, communication is fundamentally about the conveyance or transmission of a message (consciously or unconsciously) generated from one person (the sender) to another or others (the receiver). In turn, the receiver reads the message, interprets it and responds; the response in return changes so that the receiver becomes the sender and a cycle of two-way communication is initiated.

As humans, we have always communicated. Of course, communication is not just limited to man, as animals also communicate through a range of behaviours and displays. Communication has been around far longer than technology – and despite all the technology, we still continue and need to use the basic interpersonal tools with which we communicate on a person-to-person level today.

Verbal communication

Verbal communication (VC) is defined as the spoken and written word. Speech has many applications, including our private conversations or a lecture or briefing when addressing an audience, or a radio or television broadcast. Communication may be in the form of information giving, or in the giving of commands, such as a sergeant-major on a parade ground bellowing out orders. It may be in the sharing of confidences, or of problems with another such as a counsellor. Verbal communication also refers to the written word – in handwritten letters, printed in newspapers, or in emails or text messages.

Non-verbal communications

Non-verbal communications (NVCs) are those forms of communication that support or reinforce the spoken message. It is said that roughly a third of all communication is verbal, the other two-thirds non-verbal. NVCs' uses may also occur without speech and include facial expressions, a smile, a frown or the manner of a look. How we use our eyes, our body posture or positioning, the use of arms and hand gestures all convey meaning. The proximity of our body to others may evoke a sense of trusting or threat. In supporting verbal communication in speech, additionally there is paralanguage, intonations such as uh-uh, mm, or verbal prompts such as 'go on', or asking questions to further elicit information. Tone, pitch and volume of voice all add to support or reinforce a message.

The receiver

Communication works effectively if the receiver can read, interpret accurately and understand or decode the message being conveyed. If the receiver does not speak the same language communication may be lost, though it is not uncommon for a message to be understood by the use of non-verbal communication alone. Eating out in foreign countries where I have not understood the language has not totally hampered mine or the sender's ability to be understood. Accents or dialects can cause a distortion in the message as far as the receiver is concerned. At best, cultural aspects of communication can be overcome by gaining an understanding of cultural aspects of communication, although, at worst, communication if not understood by sender or receiver can cause great offence.

Other language barriers that occur are in the language of a specific profession or specialty. Computer language, for example, can be lost on many until you are in the know and understand.

In the same way, the language of healthcare can leave patients and relatives/carers ignorant of what professionals are talking about and disempowered when the language of medical terminology is alien to them. The use of abbreviations in healthcare similarly can leave people uncertain as to their meaning.

Blocks to communication, interference or noise

A crackly radio or interference is frustrating when it distorts a programme or news item. When we say we are not on the same 'wave-length' as another person, this expression originates in radio transmission and means failing to understand aspects of communication. An example of this could be youth culture – when the adults fail to understand the 'youth of today'. There may be resistance on the part of the receiver because of attitudes, judgements or ignorance, and communication may be blocked.

Other blocks to communication are failings in understanding another's values or belief systems. Attitudes can cause blocks to be put up, which may cause discrimination, or stereotyping.

What is communicated?

It has been stated that communication is about sending a message. That message could be news or an instruction. Its applications though are much broader than this. As people, we send many positive messages through our communications; our behaviours outwardly will reflect our inner thinking, or our feelings. If we are feeling good about ourselves, or having positive thoughts, this will be read though our facial expressions, our bodily behaviours, and the content of our speech: laughter, for example, is an expression of joy, contentment or maybe appreciating a joke. A smile may demonstrate positive warmth, confidence or being attracted to someone. Head nods may affirm yes or no.

Our interactions with patients will also convey positive verbal and non-verbal messages. It would be wrong to suggest that, because our patients are mentally ill, they have been stripped of all positive communications. However, the nature of their mental conditions may inhibit or distort certain aspects of positive communication giving. A patient who is severely depressed may be quite solitary, may appear low in mood in their facial expressions, may be monosyllabic in their speech and may avoid eye contact. Patients may convey many negative emotions, isolating themselves from others; a pensive or anxious look, visible shaking, a tense look or fists clenched could show they are attempting to suppress anger, while staring or avoidance of eye contact may demonstrate a threat of violence. Shouting or crying may be indicative of emotional pain.

As a mental health student nurse, there are many communication messages you will pick up from patients. As you gain experience, knowledge and skills, you will notice more about patient behaviours and communications, and will be able to interpret what these communications may mean, identifying their significance, and how they might impact on diagnosis, risk, assessment and many other aspects of mental healthcare. Content of speech may identify distortions in thinking or delusional ideas, identifying that the patient is experiencing a hallucination. It may convey anger, distress, emotional pain, apathy, lack of motivation or low mood.

Recall a moment when you met someone for the first time, whether in a social situation or at the beginning of your course. Answer these questions and record your answers for use later.

- What were your thoughts and feelings as you approached the person you didn't previously know?
- Consider your verbal and non-verbal communication: where did you look, what was your facial expression, and what were your head, hand and arm movements, body posture and positioning?
- If you were making the first move, what did you say? What opening phrase did you use? How did you combine your verbal and non-verbal communication?
- What assessment were you beginning to make of the other person?
- What if they made the first move? How did you then respond?

An outline answer is provided at the end of the chapter.

Your role in communication with mentally ill patients

If you have not worked in care environments before and particularly in mental healthcare, you will have much to learn of the nature of communication.

Patients are people, and much of their communication will be similar to our own. In fact, as health professionals, we are no different from our patients. We may have been patients ourselves or could be in the future! Our patients are people with problems arising from numerous contributing factors or causes broadly underpinned as 'nature' or 'nurture' or an interaction between the two and, subsequently, a range of responses that include maladaptive thinking and behaviours as a consequence. Some patients may convey more challenging aspects of behaviour that may vary in frequency and/or intensity, and there may be a lack of control in some patients, of anger, expressions of anxiety, distress or grief. Some communications may be bizarre and patients may describe irrational beliefs and delusional thinking. Some patients may be emotionally numbed and therefore lacking in expression.

Case study

Sarah, 19, has been admitted to the acute ward on which you are a student in your third week. She has a history of self-harm and depression, and a diagnosis of 'borderline personality disorder'. Being of roughly the same age, you are able to quickly establish a rapport with her, and have identified similar likes and interests. While on the ward, Sarah has self-harmed a couple of times, having cut her wrists with the jagged edges of a piece of glass she found out in the grounds, and concealed it. In conversation, she discloses to you that she feels that she can confide in you, that you have never been angry with her for her self-harming. She further discloses that her music teacher, with whom she used to have private piano lessons at his house between the ages of 14 continued . . . •••

> *and 18, would always touch her inappropriately and increasingly intimately. He was a good friend of her*
> *father, so Sarah could never speak out about it and no one would believe her anyway.*

Nurses will observe expressions and communications from patients and, by the same token, patients will also be observing us and how we respond to them. You will (consciously or unconsciously) be giving messages out to patients that may reflect your own inner thoughts and feelings. Communicating negative messages may be unhelpful, and we need to keep ourselves 'in check', being aware of what and how we communicate. Self-awareness of how we communicate outwardly, of what and how we project ourselves to others, is important. Our expressed warmth, a smile, a helpful comment or a compliment will all contribute to the development of positive relationships. Conversely, our judgements, negative opinions or our disapproval will be read by others. In our interactions with patients, it may at times be necessary to disguise our inner feelings or reactions: for example, if a patient explains a horrific event in his or her life in graphic detail or an allegation is made against another person, to react with shock and horror may be unhelpful, while at the same time it is important that patients are listened to and believed. We need to be aware of what could be an unconscious act, such as gasping with shock, and avoid reacting in this way, because patients will be making an assessment of us as we are assessing them. They will soon register who in the care team responds appropriately and in a kindly way to them, or those staff who are helpful or unhelpful, or those staff (and students) who they feel comfortable with and able to trust with their life stories, confidences and life experiences. This is the beginning of therapeutic communication and the process of building therapeutic relationships.

This disclosure raises the issue about what do you, the student, now do with this information given to you confidentially from a patient who felt they could trust you in opening up to you. It is vital when interacting with patients that you explain, ideally at the beginning or at an appropriate moment (being mindful that you do not wish for them to 'clam-up' or interrupt the disclosures), that you cannot keep secrets and you may need to communicate such information to your mentor or the patient's nurse/key worker as there is clearly a safeguarding issue here which will need following up by appropriately trained professionals along policy and practice guidelines. It is very likely the patient does wish the information to be known and would wish something to be done about it and hasn't previously felt safe in making that initial disclosure.

Activity 1.2   *Critical thinking*

Recall a time when you needed some form of help that you found to be a very positive experience. It could be in a course tutorial, visiting your general practitioner, enjoying a meal in a restaurant or buying clothes in a shop.

- What were you thinking immediately before you spoke with the other person?
- What behaviours did you observe in the person helping you?
- How did her or his approach to you make you feel?

An outline answer is provided at the end of the chapter.

So, having looked at communication in general, we now need to move on to look at the differences between communication and therapeutic communication.

Therapeutic communication

Being able to communicate and relate to people and their unique experience of mental distress is vital for meaningful and effective nursing intervention.
(Pearce, 2006, p97)

The therapeutic use of self: including use of personal qualities and experiences

In coming on to your mental health nurse education programme, you bring with you your life experience to date, whether you are 18 or 48 years of age. Your life has been shaped or moulded by your life experiences and you will have formed values and beliefs, and have learned positive and negative attitudes and behaviours. You will have gained achievements, have had both positive and negative life experiences, and you will have developed a sense of inner security and possibly carry with you some insecurities. What you can contribute to mental health nursing is that you will have acquired a range of communication skills, have formed healthy relationships, and will possess qualities such as compassion and a desire to care. In other words, you do not start your course as an empty vessel waiting to be 'filled up' with knowledge and skills from academics, practitioners and peers. You bring with you your own self or, to put it another way, 'your' 'self'. What your course will do for you through your patient encounters, feedback from patients, clinical and academic staff and peers, and personal reflections will further develop your self-awareness skills.

Case study

Joe, a 38-year-old man, has been admitted with depressive symptoms and has been transferred from the general hospital having taken an overdose of paracetamol capsules and antidepressant medication. It transpires that the reason for his depression is that he has had to leave the family home where he lived with his wife and stepdaughter (from his wife's first marriage) and is awaiting a court case. He has been accused of sexually molesting his stepdaughter, aged ten, which she disclosed to her schoolteacher who contacted the relevant authorities who then took action.

After handover, Jane (a first-year mental health student) is assigned to Joe to complete the admission procedure. Jane approaches Joe, who is quite communicative and easy to talk to. He does not come over as depressed; nevertheless, Jane has certain anxieties about approaching Joe.

Hearing stories from a patient who has experienced abuse or working with an abuser or an alleged abuser can challenge our values, beliefs and attitudes, and therefore our automatic thoughts and feelings may be of pity and sadness for an abused person or revulsion or disgust towards an abuser.

Concept summary: Core skills

Carl Rogers (1961) identified some core skills when working with patients and these are summarised here.

- **Genuineness**: openness and honesty in our communications, notwithstanding the need at times to suppress emotion as described above.
- **Unconditional positive regard**: in the case of Joe, it may be the act or the crime we condemn, but not the individual. Unconditional positive regard is about acceptance of the patient who has a right to care and treatment despite what he or she has done.
- **Empathy**: a number of definitions exist for the term; however, it is essentially about gaining a deep, emotional understanding of another's feelings or problems as if entering into his or her world, but not suffering his or her pain in the same way the patient would.

Activity 1.3   *Critical thinking*

Examine Jane's possible reactions to the task she has been given in the knowledge of Joe's history.

- How is it possible to achieve unconditional positive regard for Joe in the knowledge of his alleged crime?
- How may we as nurses manage our fears and judgements when confronted with such a scenario?

An outline answer is provided at the end of the chapter.

We may be shocked by what we learn of patients' histories. In cases of abuse, or while working in forensic settings, you will come across patients who have committed criminal acts at a time when mental illness was deemed to be attributable or seriously contributed to such acts taking place. Nevertheless, as nurses we have a duty to care for all patients who are admitted into the mental healthcare system with whom we come into contact and, whatever our personal feelings, we have to care for those individuals. Rationally speaking, the judicial system will have managed, or will be in the process of managing, those criminal acts and we are not required to, nor are in a position to, pass judgement on patients. We are there to care. However, our own automatic thought processes may come into play and we might be really challenged by this, be fearful and have a real problem in working with such individuals, and it is important to recognise and explore this and to gain support through clinical supervision.

In the knowledge that Joe is alleged to have committed crimes against children, it would be very easy to condemn and judge him for those acts. This poses a challenge to building a therapeutic relationship.

Therapeutic engagement is that first step in initiating the therapeutic nurse–patient relationship. Chapter 2 will explore this in more depth. The therapeutic nurse–patient relationship involves a person in need of help being connected with a person providing that help. It is about the helper giving influence or in some way facilitating a change, be that in thinking or behaviour. It involves a degree of interdependence, although within boundaries. It is about advancing the promotion of healing and change. Together you will explore the patient's feelings, and begin to understand motivations for certain behaviours in an atmosphere that promotes trust and is non-judgemental. Through the developing relationship, nurses must not be afraid of using supportive challenge or confronting a mismatch between expressed thoughts and actions.

Building partnerships and relationships

The concept of the therapeutic nurse–patient relationship is not new. As stated earlier, Peplau (1952) viewed mental health nursing on an interpersonal level and was very influential in the development of an interpersonal model of nursing still relevant today. The therapeutic nurse–patient relationship takes therapeutic engagement a stage further. Many people with mental health problems often find difficulty in initiating and sustaining relationships. It is core to the role of a mental health nurse and, as a student, you will be acquiring and developing those skills. The therapeutic nurse–patient relationship underpins much of nursing activity if it is to be effective.

There are four key interconnected values in the therapeutic relationship (O'Carroll and Park, 2007). They are power and control, partnership, boundaries and core conditions.

When you care for mentally ill patients, you will be expected to engage effectively with them in their acute stages of illness, enhance and support them through recovery, be facilitative in enhancing their well-being and enable them to move from dependence in order to regain independence to a greater or lesser degree.

Therapeutic engagement is about making a connection, an attachment, a meeting of souls as a professional carer walking a path with someone in need of care. It may feel rather strange if not a little unnatural in the beginning.

Ellis and Day (2010, in Norman and Ryrie, 2013) identified six characteristics of effective therapeutic relationships.

- **Supportive** – providing emotional and practical support.
- **Connected** – being closely connected to the feelings and experiences of the patient.
- **Facilitative** – being able to make things happen on behalf of the patient.
- **Influential** – being capable of helping the client make positive changes to his or her life.
- **Purposeful** – the nurse and patient being clear about the focus and intention of the relationship.

Ellis and Day further identify a number of qualities beneficial for students to identify and develop throughout their nursing careers. Those qualities are shown in Figure 1.1.

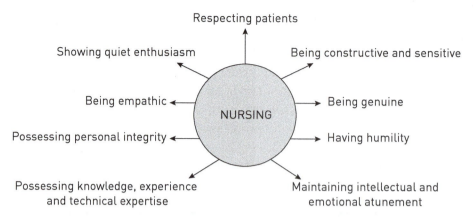

Figure 1.1: Nursing qualities (after Ellis and Day, 2010, in Norman and Ryrie, 2013)

Activity 1.4   *Reflection*

Recall a time when a friend poured her or his heart out to you with a personal or health problem.

- What did that trigger inside you?
- How did you feel?
- How did you respond?
- How did the session end? How did you know the session had brought itself to a conclusion? By you? By your friend?
- Reflecting on that conversation, identify what you did.
- What would you consider to be helpful interventions during your conversation? And reflecting afterwards?
- Is there anything that you said or did that was unhelpful?

An outline answer is provided at the end of the chapter.

A core skill you will require is that of *attentive listening*. To engage fully with your patient in attentive listening will demonstrate to him or her that you genuinely are interested. To be given that undivided attention for five minutes, ten minutes, an hour affirms to the patient that they have value and worth.

While theories as to the causation of mental ill-health are many, it is generally accepted that nature and nurture and the interface of the two are contributory factors. All too often mental illness has challenged close relationships. A failure or inability to bond from early childhood may reflect an inability to trust others in adult life. Distorted communication in families of those where an individual suffers from schizophrenia has been documented. A failure to demonstrate acceptable social skills is a common part of care-planning in developing these skills in some patients. Patients may have suffered rejection, isolation, stigmatisation and negative stereotyping from so-called 'normal' people because of deficits in how they communicate.

The purpose of therapeutic communication is how this might be improved. As a student, you will be part of a care team. Professionally, you will develop a greater sense of self and how self in relation to others will develop that therapeutic part of your being in skills development. A range of psychological interventions and skills will further equip you with the ability to effectively work with patients through using an armoury or toolkit (after Heron, 2001) of interpersonal approaches to repair such deficits; however, to engage therapeutically with patients who have a mental illness or psychiatric dysfunction demands more than just a chat over a cup of tea!

Gaining a rapport

First impressions carry great sway in how people will respond to us. This would be the same for any relationship building outside healthcare. What the other person transmits on that first engagement, at that first meeting and the transactions that follow can have a bearing on that continued relationship. If you as a student mental health nurse display warmth and openness, smile and are welcoming to patients, this approach may set the tone for how patients will see you and will assist in gaining a positive rapport with patients. Alternatively, if you are cold, aloof, controlling or judgemental, a less than helpful relationship may ensue.

Encouraging and facilitating disclosure

As part of getting to know patients, we will learn of their reason for being in the healthcare system from medical notes, referral letters, speaking with relatives and, of course, speaking with the patients themselves. As a nurse, I feel very privileged that patients have entrusted me with personal information about themselves. We dutifully must respectfully and confidentially manage the information we have about patients. In some instances, patients may freely tell us what they are happy to disclose; however, as part of the assessment of patients, we will need to go that much further in eliciting information from patients. There is a range of questioning techniques that may be used and these will be covered further in Chapter 4.

Another essential ingredient that is linked with feeling safe is the ability to form trust; for the patient, knowing that information is going to be safeguarded, particularly at a time of vulnerability and uncertainty, will determine the level of disclosure (Brown et al., 2009)

Recognising when people are anxious or in distress

Anxiety is a feeling experienced by most people at times of perceived psychological threat. This could be in sitting an exam or a driving test, and most of us would recognise those symptoms, which include a racing pulse, sweating, stomach churning and many others. It is in essence a protective mechanism and is part of the survival mechanism characterised by the 'fight or flight' response. Most of the time, we are able to control that anxiety and continue to function, and it is said that a heightened anxiety may even improve performance. Anxiety as a disorder is also one of a range of mental health disorders (APA, 2013) whereby symptoms are exaggerated. At worst, patients experience panic disorder. This may be a reaction to a phobic state. Whatever is the underlying emotion or mental disorder, mental health nurses are required to respond appropriately and therapeutically to minimise the distress. A patient in a severe panic attack may experience chest pain or a feeling of being strangled, may have an increased breathing rate or nasal flaring, may have tingling in his or her fingers (caused by reduced carbon dioxide levels due to over-breathing) and may have a feeling of impending doom or death. While this is not a serious mental illness, observing a patient in this state can be disturbing or challenging. The aim of interventions here is to bring the patient to a more relaxed state, taking control of the emotions by encouraging deep breathing. Rebreathing carbon dioxide by use of a brown paper bag is a useful technique to use when patients are experiencing tingling sensations in their fingers. Talking through the anxiety in a calm voice and offering reassurance to the patient and supporting him or her through this time is essential. Remember, though, that it is essential that you exclude angina or myocardial infarction as causes of chest pain.

Sensitivity to the impact of trauma and abuse

Many patients in the mental healthcare system experience mental health problems as a direct consequence of abuse or a traumatic event or events in their lives. Abuse has a number of forms and may be caused by neglect, physical, emotional or sexual abuse, or a combination of factors. Patients may display a range of behaviours as a consequence, which often include self-harm through wrist-cutting, acting-out behaviour, low self-esteem and depression. Suicide ideation, suicide attempts and actual suicide are common outcomes from this. Patients will often have difficulties in bonding, gaining trust, and establishing and maintaining relationships. A number of diagnoses may be given to patients who exhibit self-harming behaviours, of which borderline personality disorder is one.

Patients who have experienced trauma (and abuse may also be included here) may experience anxiety, depressive reactions and post-traumatic stress disorder (APA, 2013), for which symptoms include re-experiencing the trauma as though it were happening in the here and now, flashbacks, phobic states and mental distress. Anger responses, and misuse of alcohol and substances may be exhibited. Rather like grief, witnessing the distress can be difficult, because we may feel impotent to help (Worden, 2009).

Psychosis and therapeutic interventions

Psychoses are deemed to be the most severe of mental illnesses. Patients with psychoses may be experiencing delusional thinking or other thought disorders, may have extreme paranoia, or may be hearing voices (auditory hallucinations). They may have strange ideas or behave in very bizarre ways, which can be unnerving.

Scenario

Your mentor has assigned to your care Simon, aged 32, who suffers from paranoid schizophrenia. He had his first psychotic episode while in basic training in the army, aged 19, and was medically discharged. He has been in care ever since. He has a history of violent outbursts – he seems to be very frightened and vigilant continually, and where he sits in the day room seems to create a very large personal space around him. Other patients avoid him and staff manage him very carefully as he is prone to aggressive outbursts when afraid, although he is amenable. He is difficult to engage with, although staff comment that students have managed to build therapeutic relationships with him in the past.

You will be caring for patients with illnesses that vary in severity. Working with the acutely ill, particularly in states of psychosis, can be very challenging, even simply spending time with them, let alone engaging in therapeutic communication techniques (Bowers et al., 2010). They may present as deeply unwell, severely deluded, suspicious, hostile or aggressive. Bowers undertook research among experienced, and what were considered expert, nurses working with acutely ill psychotic patients and identified some key themes that were later put together in a monograph (Bowers et al., 2009), offering a range of interventions in managing such patients and these are described now.

Moral foundations

In this Bowers includes issues such as not ignoring the patient and, at the same time, avoiding intrusion and respecting privacy. Respect for the patient and an avoidance of harshness, even under the most challenging of circumstances, is important. Honesty with the patient around restrictions and loss of liberty and the quality of the service they received was also viewed as important.

Preparing for interaction

Preparation and knowing about the patient in advance of meeting the patient was seen as essential. Beginning to formulate a picture of the individual by reading her or his records, mental illness history and the referral letter, by speaking with relatives and people who know the patient, by careful observation and by determining the best time and location to make an approach were all considered to be positive ways of making preparation.

Being with a patient

Being with an acutely psychotic patient demands a range of approaches: engaging in therapeutic activity will have limited effectiveness, but approaches include simply sitting or being with the patient, in silence or in low-level conversation (the student having introduced him- or herself), focusing on the patient rather than his or her symptoms and engaging in some form of joint activity. In my student days, I recall meeting a very paranoid young man in his early thirties who staff had real difficulty getting alongside. He was often aggressive if staff came very close and people subsequently tended to give him a very wide berth. I considered it a breakthrough when he and I together engaged in putting the clean linen away into the linen cupboard.

Non-verbal communication, vocabulary and timing

Use of vocabulary and timing of interventions were significantly important: slow pace, slow speech, simple vocabulary repeated and careful choice of vocabulary were suggested. Tone of speech and a non-threatening manner particularly around irritable or aggressive patients were a must.

Emotional regulation

You were advised earlier not to be shocked by patient disclosures and similar good practice applies here. It was the view of the expert nurses that, to be effective, they needed to conceal their own anxiety by consciously regulating their own responses, to avoid showing anxiety when confronted with patients exhibiting overt psychotic symptoms, emotional distress or overt hostility. By the same token, it can be unnerving for a student nurse to be confronted by patients' extremes of behaviour and you will over time develop this skill while at the same time being vigilant and keeping yourself safe.

Getting things done

The daily tasks such as washing, dressing and eating require a more gentle, softly-softly approach rather than commanding patients to be compliant. It evokes a better response to be flexible, maximise choice, prompt, encourage and give positive feedback. If resistance was based on delusions, a degree of collusion was acceptable if it was balanced by the patient's need for care. Appropriate gestures for patients who were thought disordered were considered helpful.

Talking about symptoms

This was considered to be the most important by the expert mental health nurses. Hearing about patients' experiences, and accepting and validating them were essential. For patients who were withdrawn, they identified with patients the cause, worked towards an agreed care plan and used a step-by-step approach. Patients experiencing hallucinations demanded stress management techniques, distraction, bolstering and coping skills. Nurses challenged the content of delusions, and collusion was not recommended; but they adopted techniques of 'ignoring the delusions' or 'finding ways around them'.

For other forms of dysfunction, which included agitation, hyperactivity, irritability and aggression, the expert nurses recommended exercise, distraction, relaxation, avoidance of confrontation, explaining the reasons for actions and rules, negotiating advance directives and forceful containment (Bowers et al., 2009).

Chapter summary

In this chapter, we have looked at a range of concepts from basic communication theory through to therapeutic skills and the beginnings of the development of therapeutic interpersonal relationships. The chapter explored how this may be achieved given that the patients outlined are vulnerable, have a complex range of presentations and have been given psychiatric diagnoses ranging from acute anxiety states through to severe mental illness in the form of psychosis. Patients often present with disturbing personal histories, for example through their experiences of abuse, and their behaviour and emotions may be unpredictable, distressing or bizarre. Patient groups are cared for in a variety of settings, ranging from forensic secure units to the relative freedom of their own homes. Patients will span the age range from children through to old age.

Working with and caring for the mentally ill can be a very demanding profession and as a student entering into it you need to know how to discharge some of the weightiness of your patient encounters. The support of your mentors in practice, academic and pastoral tutors and clinical supervision will be explored later in the book.

Activities: brief outline answers

Activity 1.1: Reflection (page 11)

Breaking the ice with someone you have not previously met can either come very easily to us or we may find it challenging depending on the context of that meeting. It is likely that, in a split second, unconsciously we begin to scan the other person and feel comfortable in their presence and consequently respond positively towards them. We may have thoughts as to what the person thinks of us, and form opinions about what we think of the other person, such as are they kindly or domineering, or do we feel threatened by them? Does the person fit a social stereotype and do we begin to classify them as such?

Activity 1.2: Critical thinking (page 12)

Seeking help can be difficult; we may feel embarrassed that our problem feels trivial, but it is important enough to make us feel in need of help. The instant response of the person to whom we have gone for help is vital in determining how we relate to them and them to us. A helper who demonstrates a non-possessive warmth, is non-judgemental and has a genuine desire to help us will make us feel at ease, valued and important and we can begin to trust that he or she will hold information confidentially.

Activity 1.3: Critical thinking (page 14)

Jane has just learned that her patient has sexually abused a young child, a girl, and there may be a possible identification with her own gender and potential vulnerability. Jane may have feelings about her patient that he should be ashamed about what he has done, yet also feelings of anger towards him because he shows no shame; on the contrary, he is quite confident and communicative. It is quite natural to personally hold contempt for and judgement of patients who have committed crimes, particularly against children. If Jane has very strong feelings about her patient, she would be wise to speak with her mentor to seek support or explore the problem through supervision.

Activity 1.4: Reflection (page 16)

There may be an initial anxiety when people come to us in distress, whether being tearful or distraught or having angry thoughts of 'I need to stop them crying'. This is a process called *rescuing* – in stopping them crying in their distress, we are actually trying to manage *our* distress in watching them. Crying can be very therapeutic – a cathartic release allows a discharge of emotion. As the person in the helping role, it can feel quite affirming that the patient has chosen us to speak with and, while initially there may be fears about causing him or her more harm than good, gently guiding a person through his or her catharsis will give the support the person needs. Catharsis will come to a natural end. That is not to say that, after one release of emotion, that is the end of it, as catharsis can be revisited.

Further reading

Bach, S and Grant, A (2011) *Communication & Interpersonal Skills for Nurses* (2nd edition). Exeter: Learning Matters.

This is an excellent text in the series addressing communication generally across all fields of nursing and providing a useful broad background to this chapter.

Barker, P (2009) *Psychiatric and Mental Health Nursing* (2nd edition). London: Hodder-Arnold.

One of mental health nursing's leading lights on recovery and the tidal model, Phil Barker provides an all-round approach to contemporary mental health nursing practice.

Burnard, P (2001) *An Experiential and Reflective Guide for Nurses and Health Care Professionals* (5th edition). Oxford: Butterworth-Heineman.

Phil Burnard has written prolifically in the area of interpersonal skills for nurses and how nurses may develop them. This text goes that little bit deeper into how nurses further develop their practice.

McCormack, B (2010) *Person-centred Nursing*. Chichester: Wiley-Blackwell.

This text brings out the individual person-centred approach to care.

Peplau, H (1988) *Interpersonal Relations in Nursing*. London: Palgrave Macmillan.

Writing from the 1950s, Hildegard Peplau has been an extremely influential writing and nursing theorist, with her specific ground-breaking interpersonal relations model of nursing, and has informed much of the mental health nursing communication process today.

Roberts, D (2013) *Psycho-social Nursing Care: A guide to nursing the whole person*. Maidenhead: Open University Press.

On a similar theme of recognising that patients are individuals, this text stresses that our communication processes need to be individually focused.

Tee, S, Brown, J and Carpenter, D (2012) *Handbook of Mental Health Nursing*. London: Hodder-Arnold.

This text takes the reader into more depth in aspects of mental healthcare for which communication is key.

Trenoweth, S, Docherty, T and Price, I (eds) (2006) *Nursing and Mental Health Care: An introduction for all fields of practice*. Exeter: Learning Matters.

Chapter 6 of this text provides an excellent supplement to this chapter and provides an overview of communication in nursing.

Useful websites

www.england.nhs.uk/nursingvision

This website is an excellent resource for all nurses in implementing the Chief Nursing Officer's vision for nursing around compassionate care.

www.rcn.org.uk/development/health_care_support_workers/resources/RCN_Library_r esources/communicating_with_patients,_relatives_and_colleagues

This is an excellent resource provided by the RCN on communication in nursing.

www.skillsyouneed.com/interpersonal-skills.html

This is a skills-based website providing teaching and learning packages in communications skills development.

Chapter 2
What is engagement?

Wendy Turton

NMC Standards for Pre-registration Nursing Education

This chapter will address the following competency:

Domain 2: Communication and interpersonal skills

Mental health nurses must practise in a way that focuses on the therapeutic use of self. They must draw on a range of methods of engaging with people of all ages experiencing mental health problems, and those important to them, to develop and maintain therapeutic relationships. They must work alongside people, using a range of interpersonal approaches and skills to help them explore and make sense of their experiences in a way that promotes recovery.

NMC Essential Skills Clusters

This chapter will address the following ESCs:

Cluster: Care, compassion and communication

1. As partners in the care process, people can trust a newly registered graduate nurse to provide collaborative care based on the highest standards, knowledge and competence.

By the first progression point:

5. Is able to engage with people and build caring professional relationships.

By the second progression point:

6. Forms appropriate and constructive professional relationships with families and other carers.

6. People can trust the newly registered graduate nurse to engage therapeutically and actively listen to their needs and concerns, responding using skills that are helpful, providing information that is clear, accurate, meaningful and free from jargon.

By the first progression point:

3. Always seeks to confirm understanding.
4. Responds in a way that confirms what a person is communicating.
5. Effectively communicates people's stated needs and wishes to other professionals.

continued . . .

By the second progression point:

6. Uses strategies to enhance communication and remove barriers to effective communication minimising risk to people from lack of or poor communication.

Chapter aims

By the end of this chapter you should be able to:

*   describe the concept of therapeutic engagement and understand why good engagement skills are a key element of the role of the mental health nurse;
*   articulate the interpersonal dynamics of the process of engagement and the importance of increased self-awareness when initiating therapeutic relationships with service users;
*   understand how a person-centred approach to care underpins effective engagement skills;
*   apply a developed understanding of therapeutic engagement in your practice.

Effective therapeutic engagement

Coroner calls for mental health service changes after man's death.
(BBC News, 2 July 2013)

A couple of years ago, a man living with bipolar disorder, recently discharged from a Mental Health Act section, actively disengaged from contact with mental health services with tragic consequences.

Health professionals . . . can be overly protective or pessimistic about what someone with a mental health problem will be able to achieve.
(Mental Health Foundation, 2014)

Effective therapeutic engagement is the cornerstone of nursing practice; too little and the worst can happen, too much and our practice becomes paternalistic and can impede a patient's autonomy and recovery.

We need to be aware of the importance of effective therapeutic engagement for people experiencing mental health problems, and understand how to foster and sustain therapeutic engagement. As nurses we need to know how our own beliefs as well as those of service users challenge engagement, and use clinical supervision to support engagement. These are the building blocks of best practice.

Introduction

This chapter considers mental health engagement from an organisational, sociocultural and therapeutic perspective. It will show you ways you can practise effective therapeutic engagement and discusses the challenges to engagement, as well as disengagement. It reflects on social exclusion for people living with mental health problems, and considers stigmatisation within the mental health profession.

Engagement

Engagement is a key nursing process; without engagement with and by mental health service users, mental healthcare is impoverished. This is true whether the service user is engaged with a nurse or other mental health professional, or with the mental health organisation. The latter, organisational engagement, where a service user is involved in the development of services, is an agenda being pursued in the UK because, in NHS Foundation Trusts, service users are key stakeholders and so organisations have obligations and accountability to them for the quality of services they provide. The former, therapeutic engagement, is what nurses should be pursuing in routine practice because it enables us to skilfully deliver ethical and evidence-based care so that service user recovery and autonomy are supported.

Organisational engagement

These days the idea of 'organisational engagement' is built into plans for action, so as to involve service users (and other stakeholders) and give them a real say in how services are provided. We see similarities in engagement processes at different levels, for example service user to practitioner, or organisation to stakeholders – the ability to work in partnership, listen, assimilate the shared information, and work towards agreed goals focused on benefit to stakeholders. Organisational engagement is part of a change process towards viewing service users as partners in, rather than passive recipients of, care. Provided that this process gainfully uses the input of its stakeholders, then this is a laudable aim; conversely, paying lip service to any key stakeholder (e.g. service users, carers, service staff, interagency partners) diminishes the integrity of any organisation, but particularly so health providers.

If engagement fails

A recent example of devastating failures in engagement at all levels was uncovered in the Mid Staffordshire NHS Foundation Trust between 2005 and 2008, leading to failures in care that may have contributed to around three hundred deaths. The Public Enquiry into the systemic failures and subsequent neglectful care, known as the Francis Report (2013), has sparked many local initiatives (e.g. *The Listening Organisation* White Paper, Williams 2013) and national responses (e.g. *Compassion in Practice*, Commissioning Board et al., 2012) attempting to prevent similar scandalous debacles of care; all identify more effective engagement at all levels and between all stakeholders, as being paramount to supporting the consistent delivery of effective, safe and person-centred care.

Such macro-level failures are, of course, appalling, but we must not lose sight of the 'micro level' and the damage that failing to engage skilfully with our patients at a service user–practitioner level can wreak on the lives of the individuals who come into our care. As nurses we have a professional duty (NMC, 2008, 2010a) to deliver ethical and effective person-centred care, and enhancing our understanding of therapeutic engagement and our engagement skills is a significant step towards meeting this responsibility.

Engagement and nursing

The NMC *Code* (2008) does not use the word engagement; instead the approach that registered nurses are required to use with their patients in their clinical practice is to *Make the care of people your first concern, treating them as individuals and respecting their dignity* (pp3–4).

This generic prescription of behaviour includes an active focus on kindness, non-discrimination, advocacy, listening, giving information and promoting autonomy. While not specifically using the term engagement, we can see that all of these are skills that will enhance, or are enhanced by, effective therapeutic engagement.

Both the *Standards* and Essential Skill Clusters for pre-registrants (NMC, 2010a, 2010b) do use the term engagement, requiring mental health nursing students to use *a range of methods of engaging with people of all ages experiencing mental health problems, and those important to them, to develop and maintain therapeutic relationships* (NMC, 2010a, p24) and to *engage therapeutically* through developing effective communication skills (NMC, 2010b).

Engagement and policy

The way we, as mental health nurses, engage service users and develop clinically effective and ethical therapeutic relationships has become enshrined in recent UK health policies and reports. In the NIMHE (National Institute of Mental Health in England) *Guiding Statement on Recovery* (DH, 2005a) skilful engagement was defined as a key part of supporting service users through to recovery, with recovery-focused interventions being underpinned by *positive working relationships supported by good communication skills* (p5). The *Making Recovery a Reality* report by the Sainsbury's Centre for Mental Health (SCMH, now the CMH) (Shepherd et al., 2008) detailed that recovery was best supported by:

- finding and maintaining hope – believing in oneself; having a sense of personal agency; being optimistic about the future;
- re-establishment of a positive identity – finding a new identity that incorporates illness, but retains a core, positive sense of self;
- building a meaningful life – making sense of illness; finding a meaning in life, despite illness; being engaged in life;
- taking responsibility and control – feeling in control of illness and in control of life.

The Darzi Report, *High Quality Care for All* (DH, 2008a) further highlighted the importance of the service user experience within the NHS, emphasising that people need to be treated with compassion, dignity and respect; these three qualities are key features of the therapeutic relationship, which is initiated and maintained through effective therapeutic engagement.

The NICE clinical guideline for mental health service users, published in 2011 (National Collaborating Centre for Mental Health, 2012), offers evidence-based advice on ensuring a good experience of care. We need to be working in partnership with service users and their carers and families; offering help, treatment and care in an atmosphere of hope and optimism; taking the time to build trusting, supportive, empathic and non-judgemental relationships; fostering autonomy, by promoting active participation in treatment decisions and supporting self-management; and maintaining continuity of individual therapeutic relationships wherever possible. These are all undeniably essential features of mental health practice, which again can be supported through effective therapeutic engagement with service users.

And coming right up to date, *Compassion in Practice* (Commissioning Board et al., 2012), a values- and behaviour-based policy and strategy document in response to the Francis report, sets out that the *shared purpose [of] nurses, midwives and care staff [is] to deliver high quality, compassionate care, and to achieve excellent health and wellbeing outcomes* (p2). It does this through defining core values and behaviours of nursing known as the '6Cs': care, compassion, competence, communication, courage and commitment. All of the six are understood as relational constructs because each is intended to be achieved through effective therapeutic relationships with our service users; the starting point for which is – you've guessed it – effective therapeutic engagement.

Engagement to initiate and support an effective therapeutic relationship, designed to promote recovery and high-quality and safe care, includes being cognisant of these factors and many more (see Figure 2.1).

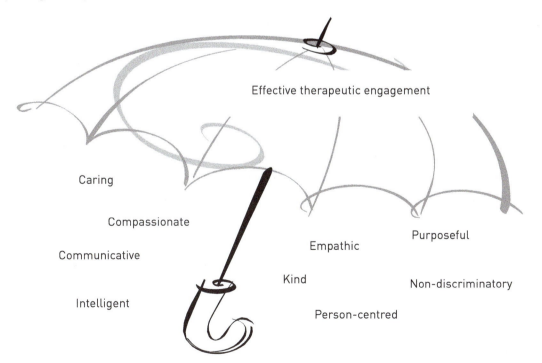

Effective therapeutic engagement

Caring

Compassionate

Communicative

Intelligent

Empathic

Kind

Person-centred

Purposeful

Non-discriminatory

Figure 2.1: Keywords under the engagement umbrella

Therapeutic engagement

Therapeutic engagement is the *process* of initiating clinical relationships with service users, with the express purpose of supporting them forward on their recovery journeys; we use engagement *skills* to develop and sustain therapeutic relationships with service users and keep them engaged in their care.

As early as 1999 the National Service Framework (NSF) for mental health stated that all care received by mental health service users should optimise engagement. Effective engagement will reduce distress, violence, suicide and self-harm, and the clinical situation will inform how we utilise engagement skills. In mental healthcare, engagement may not always be reciprocal because of the impact of the mental health problem the person is experiencing and the fact that there are times when we are empowered by statute to override the expressed wishes of a service user. But in any clinical situation, the principles of engagement do not differ; engagement must always be ethical, considered and non-discriminatory.

Engagement is an interpersonal process in which we are developing a particular type of relationship that operates with different rules from those of personal relationships. When we engage therapeutically we are connecting with explicit responsibilities of care towards that person and we have obligations placed on us because of our professional role; we are making a deliberate connection that has a therapeutic aim.

The aims of engagement include assessment, developing a shared understanding, and planning how to manage the person's experience. Engagement skills are then further used to develop a therapeutic relationship, through which care is delivered and progression towards personal recovery is supported. Effective engagement skills promote trust and safety, and serve to reduce distress, making personal difficulties more accessible to change. Acceptance and genuineness by the mental health nurse during engagement can impact positively on the sense of self that the service user has at that time, further promoting a sense of safety and recovery.

We mostly engage with people verbally and verbal therapeutic engagement skills are very different from general conversation skills. In a conversation, there is frequently no predetermined aim; it is usually mutual and balanced, is informed by life experiences or occurrences, is spontaneous and can happen anywhere; furthermore, confidentiality is not a prime concern – we simply 'chat' about things. In mental healthcare, every encounter should be therapeutic. Therapeutic engagement *does* have a predetermined aim; the focus of the interchange is the service user, it is usually planned (although do not discount the importance of naturally occurring opportunities for engagement), the environment in which it happens is important, and confidentiality is paramount. Moreover, therapeutic engagement is informed by theory and bounded by our professional codes.

Preparing for effective therapeutic engagement

The journey to learning how we engage begins with learning how to prepare ourselves to engage with those in our care, and the basis of this learning is to develop your generic psychotherapeutic skills. A framework that can be usefully drawn on to support this learning is the Improving Access to Psychological Therapies (IAPT) Cognitive Behavioural Therapy (CBT) Competencies Framework (Roth and Pilling, 2007). This framework is organised into five domains, four of which are specific to CBT competencies, but the first domain details generic psychotherapeutic competencies *needed to relate to people and to carry out any form of psychological intervention* (p7), of which engagement is one. The framework notes that skills need to be built in three areas: your knowledge of mental health, skills in building a therapeutic alliance, and skills in assessment. Take a moment to reflect on Table 2.1.

Area	Competencies
Knowledge	• knowledge and understanding of mental health problems • knowledge of, and ability to operate within, professional and ethical guidelines • knowledge of a model of therapy • ability to understand and employ the model in practice
Building a therapeutic alliance	• ability to engage client • ability to foster and maintain a good therapeutic alliance, and to grasp the client's perspective and 'world view' • ability to deal with emotional content of sessions • ability to manage endings
Assessment	• ability to undertake generic assessment (relevant history and identifying suitability for a intervention) • ability to make use of supervision

Table 2.1: Generic psychotherapeutic competencies (Roth and Pilling, 2007)

The Roth and Pilling (2007) framework further describes the following factors that can support effective and ethical therapeutic engagement:

* engender trust;
* be warm and genuine;
* show concern and confidence;
* know the boundaries of professional relationships;
* develop rapport;

- acknowledge emotional experiences;
- adjust the level of discussion to match the person's needs and capabilities at that moment;
- avoid negative interpersonal behaviours in yourself.

For mental health nursing practice this framework informs on the preparatory conditions of engaging with service users and their families and friends. Developed knowledge of mental health problems, both from a theoretical and a lived experience perspective, is an influential factor of our chosen engagement style. The list then tells us the practical skills we need to be using in order to engage effectively.

Helpful questions to ask ourselves

For the person we intend to engage with, what do we know about the mental health problem that he or she is experiencing? What does our knowledge about his or her particular experience tell us about how we can best engage? What interpersonal issues may be present given the person's mental health difficulties? How do we need to modify our approach so that our engagement is successful? We will need to ensure that our chosen approach and aim is both ethical and within our professional code. The following case study illustrates how preparation enhances engagement.

Case study

Debbie is a 37-year-old woman who is being supported in the community by the Hospital@Home Service. Debbie has been living with depression for about five years, and has been used to managing with community support from her Community Psychiatric Nurse (CPN). Over the past week Debbie has become increasingly depressed, getting out of bed is a challenge and her self-care has become poor. Her husband and friends have rallied round to look after the two children, Freya, five, and Tom, who is just three years old, so there are no current safeguarding issues. The focus of care is to provide increased support in Debbie's home environment to prevent her admission to a psychiatric hospital; therapeutic engagement and continual assessment are necessary features of this input.

Activity 2.2   *Critical thinking*

You are one of the H&H team who are visiting Debbie four times across each day, for the next four days. This is your first visit to Debbie on day 2 of her support from the H&H team; your aim is to assess her mental state and psychosocial functioning with a view to supporting crisis reduction and promoting recovery. Engagement skills are emphasised in such care episodes to help Debbie utilise the care that is being offered.

- What do you know about depression?
- What interpersonal challenges might Debbie's current experience of depression cause for engagement?
- How will you use these two areas of knowledge to inform your engagement style?

An outline answer is provided at the end of the chapter.

Engagement and the person-centred approach

Therapeutic engagement is rooted in a person-centred approach, an approach that underpins best nursing practice. This approach stems from the work of Carl Rogers (1957) and his three central principles support us as nurses to engage effectively and provide recovery-focused care to all of our service users because they support a compassionate and optimistic view of all people and drive the need to connect therapeutically with those in our care. Rogers believed that all people, once extreme problematic mental health states have been eased, are basically rational, cooperative and capable of recognising the need for and working towards change, these characteristics being released through a relationship that is therapeutic. Rogers' person-centred approach described three factors needed to engage and develop a therapeutic relationship and enable the service user to move towards change: warmth, empathy and genuineness.

Rogers noted that engagement happens in stages, which is useful to reflect on when our attempts at engaging someone do not go according to plan. Engagement can begin with defensiveness and resistance to change, moving through to increased flexibility and the development of a reflective focus on psychological issues, and culminating in a more positive sense of self and self-directed change. Patience and flexibility are professional virtues here, along with persistence – reminding yourself of the challenges that the service user is currently living with will help you retain empathy and commitment.

How to engage

While we meet each service user as an individual, there are a number of skills and factors to be aware of in each engagement opportunity. Table 2.2 presents a list of practical skills we need to use when engaging with our service users. Take some time to reflect on them as they are crucial to skill development and better practice.

Why are you attempting to engage?

Knowing why we are engaging and why we are initiating a therapeutic relationship is very important. Sometimes engagement needs to happen very quickly in order to manage immediate risk, and our priorities and behaviours will inevitably be different from when we are building longer-term relationships. However, it is important to stick to the principles of engagement to ensure that you are behaving ethically and professionally, and in a style that supports effective therapeutic engagement even in crisis situations. You will still be able to use skills from Table 2.2; indeed you should be using them in all therapeutic encounters, and in adhering to these principles you will increase the possibility of de-escalating a situation and reducing risk.

When an opportunity for non-crisis or post-crisis engagement is available, it is crucial that you keep in mind that your role with the service user is to support bio-psychosocial recovery. This focus will enable us to take an holistic approach to care. It is insufficient to recovery to merely ascertain if people are adherent to their medication regime or attending appointments. Engaging someone in mental healthcare needs to include all aspects of the person's experience. Time invested in effectively engaging someone and getting to know him or her while developing a trusting, respectful relationship will allow for the service user to share with you salient aspects of

Make and prioritise time to engage.	Find an appropriate place to meet.
Know beforehand why you are planning to engage.	Be respectful, courteous, patient and appropriate.
Respect the person's privacy and protect his or her dignity.	Express general understanding for the person's distress or situation, and be genuine.
Make good eye contact, and be aware of your posture – body language is very powerful.	Use 'low expressed emotion', i.e. be warm and don't criticise.
Be appropriately flexible.	Be honest and transparent.
Be compassionate, kind and empathetic.	Be available, reliable and consistent.
Use active listening and try not to rely on your assumptions or preformed beliefs; don't interpret or assume – ask the question!	Be aware of the person's mental health problem and take into account how it may impact on the engagement process.
Use yourself as a guide – engage in a manner that you would want your nearest and dearest engaged with if they were mental health service users.	

Table 2.2: Practical tips: how to engage

his or her experience and develop a shared understanding that then enables you to support the person more meaningfully in his or her personal recovery.

The desired outcome for therapeutic engagement and the initiation of a therapeutic relationship concerns the promotion of a shared understanding, the reduction of distress or risk, providing a sense of safety, offering a chance for reflection and guiding towards goal attainment or recovery.

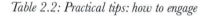

Case study

Doreen has been involved with mental health services for ten years. She lives with recurrent depression, which has led to a pattern of inpatient care for about four weeks once every 18 months. The purpose of the admissions is to stabilise mood, manage risk to self and self-neglect, kick-start an improvement in her mood, and reconsider her medication; the admissions are usually successful in doing this.

continued . . .

In between admissions Doreen recovers from the overwhelming episode, resumes her everyday life, but then slides back into overwhelming low mood. It is a cycle that is very disruptive to Doreen's life. She wants it to change but believes that it is too late to do anything about it now. She cannot hold down a long-term job, and now even struggles to get short-term employment because of her mental health history. During her 'out of hospital' phases, Doreen is seen infrequently because she is not considered high risk during this phase and her care plan is about watchful waiting for worsening depression.

It is shown that, while initial onset of depression is often linked to an external trigger event such as relationship breakdown or some sort of experience of loss or failure, further episodes can be triggered by internal events such as negative thoughts or a heightened reaction to a bad couple of days. Often people with recurrent depression notice signs of naturally occurring lower mood states (which we all are susceptible to) but understandably react to them by fearing or believing that they signify the return of their depression. This reaction increases negative thinking, which fuels a further drop in mood; this, when linked to behavioural changes such as withdrawing, can create a vicious cycle into depression.

In the above case study, the existing care plan did not prioritise knowledge about depression, engagement, person-centred care or the development of a therapeutic relationship through which to support change and recovery. While it does provide safety when Doreen's mood is at its worst, it neither breaks the cycle of 'admission–recovery–admission' for Doreen nor increases her understanding of depression and her ability to contribute to staying well.

Case study

Prior to Doreen's last inpatient discharge, the Community Team changed their approach following an agreement with Doreen that they would support her to address the pattern of recurrent admissions and so promote a more stable life with the possibility of longer-term achievements. The plan agreed was that Doreen would work with a CPN on a weekly basis initially to develop a bio-psychosocial understanding of her experience of depression, the aim of which would be to support Doreen to develop her sense of control over her recurrent experiences of depression and achieve greater stability in her mood and her life. Longer-term involvement would be to support Doreen in recognising her mood changes and actively taking steps to prevent a descent into depression.

When we reflect on this case study we can see that the new plan prioritises promoting recovery and providing hope; it is person-centred as it places Doreen's wishes for staying well at the heart of the plan. The plan is also supported by knowledge about depression. The progress of the new care plan is achieved by prioritising therapeutic engagement with Doreen so that an effective therapeutic relationship can be developed, and this is used as the vehicle to undertake the collaborative psychosocial work required to change Doreen's pattern of depression.

Case study

Doreen has not been an inpatient for three years and was discharged from the Community Team back to her GP nine months ago. She received weekly input for 12 weeks, followed by monthly meetings and telephone contact with her CPN in between meetings. Doreen had a change of CPN during this time and this was eased by two joint meetings between the incoming and outgoing nurses and Doreen to ensure continuity in approach and strengthen engagement with the service, the care plan and the new nurse.

There are times when we cannot use verbal engagement and it is important not to underestimate the importance of non-verbal engagement with those who are unable to participate in a therapeutic discourse. Sitting with, just being with someone – *the way we are present* (Rogers, 1957), bringing a drink or snack, or simply being present for someone not able to actively converse, begins an engagement process and initiates a therapeutic relationship. The following scenario encourages you to think about engagement from the inside out.

Scenario

Step into Rose's shoes. You are Rose, and have been an inpatient on the local acute psychiatric unit for three days now. You feel awful, very low in mood, and you just don't want to talk to anyone – it feels like it's just too much effort at the moment. To be honest, everything is too much at the moment, and you find yourself staying in your bed as long as you are allowed to, not washing, brushing your hair, eating, or even bothering to make a drink for yourself. You are feeling hopeless, your depression has come back and you just can't seem to pick yourself up from this episode. You can't seem to think clearly, it's like thinking through mud. You are aware that there are a few really disturbed patients on the unit at the moment who seem to need a lot of time from the staff, so it seems best not to bother anyone and just keep yourself to yourself.

Activity 2.3   *Critical thinking*

Imagine you are Rose.

- What challenges does your current mental health experience bring to the engagement process?
- Why do mental health nursing staff need to engage with you?

Now look at the other side of the engagement partnership.

- Given the ward environment and Rose's current mindset, how might you begin to engage with Rose to develop an effective therapeutic relationship that offers therapeutic benefit to her at this time?

An outline answer is provided at the end of the chapter.

The complexity of engaging

If only engagement was as simple as following a list of 'how to' skills! Unfortunately, effective therapeutic engagement is a complex activity. And in spite of all the skills at our disposal, the most powerful and effective therapeutic tool we have is ourselves; we are the vehicle for effective engagement along with all of our attendant beliefs, experiences and knowledge.

Engagement, as we have agreed, is relational, it is between people and that means that both parties in the process bring with them a number of factors that will impinge on the engagement process (see Figure 2.2).

When we engage, both we and the other person arrive with various pre-existing beliefs and life experiences: these may match or not; they may be helpful or not. The service user has the

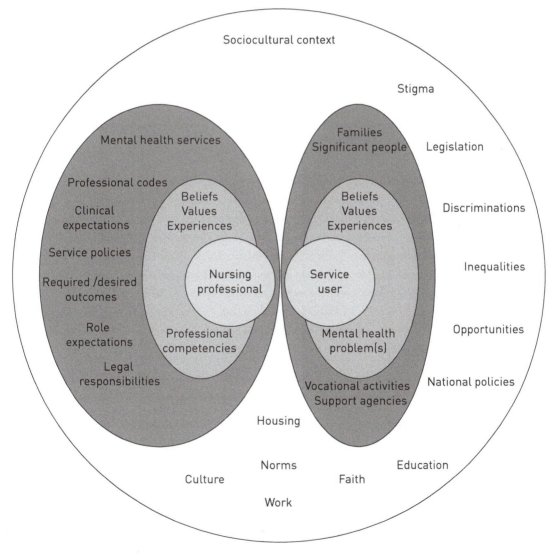

Figure 2.2: The complexity of interpersonal engagement

additional disadvantage of his or her current problematic mental state impacting on the ability to engage therapeutically with you. For both parties, any meeting will take place within a sociocultural context that sets a stage for attitudes, treatments and possibilities. The mental health nurse also brings the obligations of her or his professional and service responsibilities. All of these factors determine the quality of the therapeutic relationship we develop.

Engagement is an interpersonal activity – it happens between people, and our interpersonal styles are exposed by the activity: how we talk, what we say, and how we say it. We cannot expect that the other person will alter his or her style or beliefs to suit ours, although people do often become more matched as the relationship develops. We are not always aware of personal factors that might be troublesome to good engagement, so we have to develop a reflective approach to ourselves and our style of mental health nursing – one that becomes a constant learning opportunity during our careers. The most effective way of learning is to question ourselves about what it is that we have been doing, and what the outcome might have been, or was – if so, or if not, why? We can ask ourselves what the service user could have perceived or experienced from us, and how we think we could change in order to achieve a more desirable outcome. The most effective forum for reflection is good clinical supervision, but as this is often unavailable, our professional responsibility is to do this task for ourselves – a constant evaluation, with remedial action if required. The following scenario illustrates the power of beliefs in engagement.

Scenario

Damien is 23, and lives alone in social housing, having spent his teenage years in local authority care. Damien has been an informal inpatient for two months following a Section 2 admission under the Mental Health Act. Prior to admission Damien had been reported to the police on three occasions by his neighbours for behaviour perceived to be threatening, unreasonable and antisocial. Damien describes this time as a phase of heavy drinking alternating with frequent use of legal highs, particularly 'Salvia'. At the time of admission Damien had been persuaded to visit his GP by a friend who was worried by Damien's mood swings and anxiety. Damien was also struggling to maintain his job with a local builder because of his unreliability and temper. On admission Damien was verbally threatening to all involved, but oscillated between tears and expressions of despair with threats to self-harm, anger and threats to hurt those he saw 'interfering' in his life, and worries and anxiety about his current experience and fear of being out of control.

Damien has responded well to the calming influence of inpatient care and is working towards discharge. He has worked well with the nursing team and has been observably supportive of some of his fellow patients.

Two nights ago, however, Damien left the ward with two other inpatients and visited the local pub. From there he went on to a local night club, returning at 10 o'clock the following day, having spent the night sleeping rough in the inpatient unit grounds. Since return, Damien has been tearful and withdrawn; staff are overtly vexed by his behaviour. His psychiatrist has suggested that Damien is discharged immediately for his poor behaviour. In order to resolve the situation someone needs to re-engage with Damien to find out more about what happened, so that decisions about continuing care can be negotiated.

Activity 2.4   *Critical thinking*

- What beliefs and associated emotions could be present in the nursing team that could impact negatively on engagement with Damien?
- What beliefs would be more helpful to hold when re-engaging with Damien so that an effective therapeutic relationship can be developed?
- What beliefs and associated emotions might Damien have about himself, the incident and nursing staff's reactions that could create challenges to engagement?
- How might you initiate re-engagement with Damien?

An outline answer is provided at the end of the chapter.

Disengagement

Disengagement from mental health services in the UK averages around 30 per cent (O'Brien et al., 2009). This means that three in ten patients involved with mental health services will break off contact. The reason for such disengagement appears to fall into one of three categories: problems with the service user, the practitioner or the service ethos of care (Priebe et al., 2005). Service user factors in disengagement include ethnicity, poverty and age, and clinical factors such as insight, substance misuse and forensic history. Further factors include a desire to be independent, a poor therapeutic relationship and the deleterious psychosocial effects of medication (Priebe et al., 2005).

What do we mean when we say that a service user is disengaging? It is easy to conclude that someone has disengaged from mental healthcare if they consistently avoid you, or state clearly that they no longer wish for your support. We can see the disengagement as either appropriate or inappropriate depending on our clinical judgement of the mental state of the service user. If our informed perception is that the disengagement is inappropriate, we may pursue assertive re-engagement, which may include using statutory means to enforce engagement with services, such as Community Treatment Orders. But there are less obvious occurrences that are harder to determine. Is it disengagement to disagree with a proffered treatment protocol? Are you engaged if you are not in concordance with recommended treatment? Can a therapeutic relationship be sustained if the service user is choosing courses of action that are not in alignment with his or her care plan? These questions fall into the ethical domain of mental health nursing practice and our answers can indicate our attitudes towards mental health and its care.

It is a truth that enhancing engagement will reduce the possibility of disengagement because effective therapeutic engagement is inclusive and collaborative and respects the position of the service user, while being realistic about risk. But it is also true that some people simply choose to disengage from mental healthcare. When service users disengage we understandably do, and should, spend time thinking about why it happened as well as what steps we should take to re-engage. Sometimes our assumptions can be ill-informed as they are developed from our one-sided, albeit clinically informed, perspective and influenced by our own beliefs – we can never know for sure unless we are able to ask the service user and have a sufficiently good therapeutic relationship for her or him to be honest with us. Service user resentment towards mental health service interventions and lack of insight are often assumed to drive disengagement, but the key issues seem to be autonomy and identity: *Disengagement was often a result of the struggle against loss of autonomy and identity as a part of the experience of mental illness* (Priebe et al., 2005, p442).

In mental health, issues of autonomy, person-centred care, advocacy, risk and capacity will inevitably present challenges to engagement. Autonomy can be compromised by a sense of powerlessness engendered in therapeutic relationships, and not being listened to can often lead to a fundamental breakdown in the therapeutic relationship and consequently to disengagement. Autonomy can be supported within the therapeutic relationship through increased collaboration, supported responsibility taking, active listening and having a realistic and shared understanding of the service user's current capabilities; this, of course, is supplemented by transparency in risk management. Furthermore, increasing empathy, rather than sympathy, will discourage developing an overly paternalistic style.

Case study

Michael has been under the care of mental health services for four years now, meeting regularly with his CPN and less so with his psychiatrist. Michael lives with a diagnosis of bipolar disorder and has made good progress since his last manic episode 18 months ago. He has re-enrolled at university and is managing his mood and lifestyle in a positive way. Michael has developed a good relationship with his Community Care Team over the years and used their support to good effect. On the most recent meeting with his CPN, Michael shares that he has reduced his medication; he says he feels that he is 'better' now and is optimistic about continuing to manage his mood through psychosocial interventions.

The medication makes him tired and overweight, neither of which he wants to feel at this time in his life when things are back on track.

Michael's CPN is cautious; he remembers Michael's chaotic lifestyle before, when his mood was disregulated, and worries about how vulnerable Michael became to exploitation by other people. He is concerned that Michael's sense of optimism is heralding an overly high mood state. But he also knows that Michael has been working very hard to learn to manage his bipolar experience and that succeeding in returning to university and a 'normal, not ill' life has been Michael's goal.

Activity 2.5   *Critical thinking*

- What challenges does Michael's situation bring to therapeutic engagement and the therapeutic relationship?
- How does his case highlight issues of autonomy and identity?
- How would you, as Michael's CPN, develop the therapeutic relationship to support both autonomy and risk?
- What features of the therapeutic relationship would you enhance to prevent disengagement?

An outline answer is provided at the end of the chapter.

Stigmatisation by mental health professionals

For mental health nurses, an important dimension noted in the Royal College of Psychiatrists' *Mental Health and Social Inclusion: Making psychiatry and mental health services fit for the 21st century* position paper is the *low expectations of mental health professionals as to what people with mental health problems can achieve* (2009, p11). This professional stigmatisation supplements societal stigma and creates self-stigma, whereby people living with mental health problems come to believe the stigmatised attitudes of others and perceive themselves as a personification of the stigmatised beliefs.

There is an assumption that mental health professionals are somehow immune to stigmatising others, but this robustly appears not to be the case. It has unfortunately been shown that contact with mental health services is perceived as the second most stigmatising experience for people experiencing mental health problems and for their families.

Stigmatising attitudes influence the quality of interactions with service users and negatively influence professional judgements and behaviours. Stigmatising attitudes develop from poor understanding, and from poor experience of the treatment of, or interaction with, people experiencing particular mental health problems, and lead to a distancing from the service user; this distancing maintains stigmatising attitudes. Such attitudes affect engagement and the therapeutic relationship that is developed; by impacting on these processes, such prejudicial or ill-informed beliefs will ultimately impact on psychosocial outcomes for the service user.

Case study

Kevin has lived with psychosis since he was 18. He lives alone in a council flat and has two close friends living nearby. His life is very disrupted by his enduring experience of psychosis; he continues to hear voices and can become very paranoid. His self-care is not very good; he eats mainly takeaway food and often makes one meal last a few days, leaving the food in his living room rather than storing it appropriately. He drinks a little too much alcohol, he smokes 30 cigarettes a day and he takes no exercise. He spends most of his day in his armchair, thinking or listening to music. Kevin has known many CPNs over the years – some he got on with, others less so. He is adherent to a complex medication regime of combined antipsychotics. Kevin will not leave his block of flats so all meetings have to be at his own home.

Enduring psychosis brings with it primary and secondary problems. Kevin's continuing primary symptoms (hearing voices and paranoia) continue to cause him distress and restrict the life he leads. His secondary symptoms include side effects of his medication and physical health problems from his enforced lifestyle. People with enduring psychosis are at high risk of serious physical health problems and die on average ten years earlier than they would otherwise.

It is necessary for the mental health team to engage with Kevin so as to deliver care to optimise his (mental and physical) health, but Kevin does not see the need for assertive engagement as he just wants to live as he does and not be unnecessarily interfered with.

continued . . .

Engaging Kevin and developing a therapeutic relationship that enabled the mental health team to take the best care of Kevin took time and patience. Kevin was referred to the Assertive Outreach team, so that more than one member of the team was involved in developing the relationship with him. Early visits to Kevin's home were weekly and lasted for about half an hour; the nurse sat with Kevin, chatting about everyday things, his musical interests and football, encouraging Kevin to talk, and enquiring if there was anything that the team could do to help. Behavioural tasks were shared to encourage engagement and trust; one visit involved helping to mend an indoor washing line in Kevin's bathroom, another involved helping Kevin set up his stereo system properly. These activities enabled conversations to happen without the stress that just sitting together caused Kevin. Over the weeks, the persistence, warmth, patience and focus of the nurses paid off and Kevin became able to accept enquiries about his health and expressions of concern about his well-being, and it opened a channel of communication between the nurses and Kevin. Kevin was finally able to accept supported visits to his GP and became properly treated for his physical health concerns. This was important as, although mental health staff had concerns that he might be ill, they had no evidence. Engaged in this care regime, both Kevin's mental health and his physical condition improved and he became more active and happier, and his psychosis reduced. Along with this improvement Kevin became more engaged with life, his self-care improved and his social contact increased. Nurses had to prioritise engagement in the face of indifference and sometimes annoyance from Kevin. Skills of warmth, empathy, compassion and patience had to be utilised consistently, and care had to be offered without compromising Kevin's autonomy.

Social exclusion and mental health: supporting wider engagement

Social inclusion is societal participation enabling access to the opportunities available in that society. Mental health problems can lead to social exclusion; if we are socially excluded we are disengaged from society and all its opportunities and roles, and such disengagement is often caused and perpetuated by a society's included people – *non-participation arising from constraint, rather than choice* (Royal College of Psychiatrists, 2009, p1). The causes of social exclusion can be poverty, difference or living outside sociocultural norms. Interestingly for mental health, social exclusion appears to be a result of stigma and is independent of material wealth or other causal factors (Morgan et al., 2007).

For mental health, social exclusion has in recent years become a ubiquitous term for the social disadvantage that both results from, and is a causal factor for, poor mental health. In England and Wales in 1997, the then Labour government set up the Social Exclusion Unit to report on all aspects of societal exclusion and inform government action on reducing it; the Unit was abolished in 2010 by the Coalition government. In 2004, the Unit produced its *Mental Health and Social Exclusion* report; adults with mental health problems were noted to be one of the most socially excluded groups in society with only 25 per cent in paid employment despite the majority wanting to work. There was shown to be a dearth of leisure activities and high levels of isolation, isolation being a significant risk factor in suicide and relapse. The report notes:

Mental health problems are estimated to cost the country over £77 billion a year through the costs of care, economic losses and premature death. Early intervention to keep people in work and maintain social contacts can significantly reduce these costs. Once a person has reached crisis point, it is much more difficult and costly to restore their employment and social status.
(2004, p3)

The causes of such social exclusion were seen to be stigma, discrimination, low expectations by healthcare professionals, and barriers to accessing community resources. The report recommended addressing stigma and discrimination against mental health nationally, and offering supported social inclusion.

In 2009, the aforementioned position paper by the Royal College of Psychiatrists, *Mental Health and Social Inclusion: Making psychiatry and mental health services fit for the 21st century*, called for a socially inclusive approach to underpin the practice of all mental health professionals and to drive service culture and design. A key part of this is being genuinely adherent to a person-centred approach with service users, and promoting cultural change in attitudes and practice within services; care needs to strive to be recovery-oriented and delivering *socially inclusive outcomes.*

Fostering social inclusivity has become an emphatic antidote to social exclusion, but increasing participation in, and acceptance by, society is a complex task. It cannot be achieved by simply repositioning an excluded person's life into society, as society has to be open to that individual, granting him or her equal access, respect and non-prejudicial treatment. Equally, the excluded individual has to embrace re-entry into society with all its attendant challenges, including persisting stigma, social cruelty and potential 'failure' to re-engage successfully. And while inclusivity is a magnanimous aim, being perceived as needing supported social inclusion can, in itself, be stigmatising. Mental health professionals have to walk this tightrope – how do you promote the social inclusion of a service user by supporting her or his engagement with the wider socio-political context, and so acting to moderate the deleterious effects of social exclusion, without further stigmatising or creating exposure to potentially harmful social responses from others? The lived experience of people with mental health problems notes how societal responses contribute to excluding them from social activities and social spaces.

A key national document from 2004, which is still relevant to practice today, *The Ten Essential Shared Capabilities* (Hope, 2004), underpinned the development of a socially inclusive healthcare workforce. This document was honed in 2007 to create a series of principles for inclusive nursing practice (DH, 2007). These principles are important as they define a way of engaging with service users to promote socially inclusive outcomes. Ethical partnership working adhering to a person-centred model and respecting diversity, equality and challenging inequalities should be the agenda for all practice to enable effective assessment of needs and strengths to be undertaken, aimed at promoting recovery. The mental health nurse needs to be promoting both safety and positive risk taking, and this can only realistically be done effectively and safely if the service user is well engaged and a robust therapeutic relationship exists between nurse and service user. Further, the nurse should 'make a difference' and this is probably the bottom line – that there should be a professional commitment to engagement in and beyond the care of people who are in need of support and treatment from mental health services.

Chapter summary

Therapeutic engagement is the cornerstone of mental health nursing practice and effective therapeutic engagement is the aim of every encounter with mental health service users. Effective therapeutic engagement reduces distress and risk, and supports personal recovery. Engagement skills need to be used in every situation requiring a therapeutic connection, regardless of time available or nature of encounter. Mental health nurses need to be active in engaging service users in a wider context beyond immediate clinical need. Pre-existing attitudes and beliefs can create challenges for effective engagement. Stigmatisation still exists in the mental health profession, is detrimental to recovery and confirms societal stigma. As a mental health nurse you are in a position to make a difference.

Activities: brief outline answers

Answers are intended to support your reflections and participation in the activities and offer direction to your learning.

Activity 2.1: Reflection (page 28)

You may have listed: promoting recovery, developing understanding, ethical, professional, theory-led, relationship, listening, society, organisational, patience, policy, best practice, beliefs, attitudes, actions, reduces distress, low expressed emotion, safety.

Activity 2.2: Critical thinking (page 30)

Depression is experienced as low mood and is associated with overwhelming negativity and poor motivation and energy levels. Self-care is usually impoverished and the ability to care for others diminished. Activity levels are low. At its worst, depression is associated with risk of harm to the self. Cognitive abilities are impaired, leading to poor concentration and memory. Interpersonal communication is challenging, and speech rate and content are impoverished. Knowing this, you will need to alter your engagement style to accommodate to Debbie's cognitive impairments and low mood. Low expressed emotion, chunking information into smaller pieces, and just being with Debbie, will all enhance engagement and so reduce risk and promote recovery. You may need to support Debbie in managing the practical tasks she needs to accomplish to continue her role as best she can in caring for her family; engaging with her supporters will be helpful.

Activity 2.3: Critical thinking (page 34)

Rose is depressed and withdrawn. She is not creating a crisis situation that demands engagement, nor does she actively seek engagement with staff as she does not believe that she is important enough to be engaged with. Engagement is required because Rose's mood state is leading to self-neglect and her withdrawal may lead to a worsening of her mood. As nurses, we probably need to engage Rose through supporting her self-care, by offering Rose a drink, helping her to sit in the dining area and eat a little food, or maybe offering to support Rose to bathe. These behavioural activities can be preliminary engagement interventions that initiate a relationship that then allows for more recovery-focused interventions. Just being with Rose, sitting with her, or seeking her out can also develop the therapeutic relationship. Rose needs to see that her 'quiet' needs are as important as those of others who are expressing more visible needs to nursing staff.

Activity 2.4: Critical thinking (page 37)

You might have thought about: anger stemming from feeling let down by Damien, frustration stemming from Damien making poor choices again, dismissiveness stemming from the affirmation of your negative attitude that 'people like Damien never change'. You will need to be thinking more about not punishing Damien but rather helping him to understand why this situation arose, what the costs were, and how he might develop the skills to be less vulnerable to such temptations in the future. Damien might be feeling angry in anticipation of a punitive attitude from the staff; he may be feeling angry with himself and so finding re-engagement difficult because he has a negative view of himself; he may be feeling sad that this has happened and wanting help to put things right. Re-engaging Damien needs to be approached carefully so that Damien does not fear punishment or abandonment. Being transparent and focused with Damien about what you have to talk about and why is useful so that critical comments are neither leaking from the staff team members nor being misperceived by Damien. Avoiding being paternalistic is also important; engaging Damien in a collaborative discussion of the event is the way forward.

Activity 2.5: Critical thinking (page 38)

You may have thought about: the dilemma of medication adherence for staying well and Michael's needs to be physically fit and active at this time of his life. Michael, as a young person, is vulnerable to perceiving care as paternalistic and impinging on his independence. Michael is attempting to create an identity beyond his illness and persisting in over-nurturing care may cause frustration and disengagement. You own responsibility to keep Michael safe and well in spite of his current perspective of being able to maintain wellness while stopping his medication. Engagement needs to support collaborative and transparent care. Risk issues need to be discussed and support offered to Michael to allow his wishes to be supported while managing potential risk of breakdown. Working with Michael to increase his awareness and understanding of his illness will be imperative to develop a realistic yet acceptably autonomous care plan.

Further reading

Ballatt, J and Campling, P (2011) *Intelligent Kindness: Reforming the culture of healthcare.* London: Royal College of Psychiatrists.

This is an interesting read on developing a healthcare environment that enables compassionate care to be delivered.

Bowers, L, Brennan, G, Winship, G and Theodoridou, C (2009) *Talking with Acutely Psychotic People.* London: City University. Available online at www.iop.kcl.ac.uk/iopweb/blob/downloads/locator/l_436_Talking.pdf (accessed 14 June 2013).

This is an exceptional study detailing how best to engage with people experiencing acute psychosis.

Commissioning Board, Chief Nursing Officer and DH Chief Nursing Adviser (2012) *Compassion in Practice.* Available online at www.england.nhs.uk/wp-content/uploads/2012/12/compassion-in-practice.pdf (accessed 12 June 2013).

This national nursing report, in response to the Francis report, details how nursing practice must change to support the delivery of compassionate, safe and ethical care.

Hamilton, S, Research and Innovations Teams, Rethink (2010) *Report for NMC on Nursing Skills for Working with People with a Mental Health Diagnosis.* London: Rethink. Available online at www.nmc-uk.org/Documents/Consultations/RPNE/Report%20for%20Nursing%20and%20Midwifery%20Council%20on%20nursing%20skills%20for%20working%20with%20people%20with%20a%20mental%20health%20diagnosis.pdf (accessed 14 June 2013).

This is an excellent report detailing recommendations for best practice by mental health nurses.

LeCroy, C and Holschuh, J (eds) (2009) *First Person Accounts of Mental Illness and Recovery: Case examples of living with a mental disorder.* Hoboken, NJ: Wiley.

It is always worth supplementing your knowledge by reading first-person accounts. This book provides some thought-provoking accounts of living with mental health problems that will support your practice development.

National Collaborating Centre for Mental Health (2012) *Service User Experience in Adult Mental Health.* Leicester and London: British Psychological Society and Royal College of Psychiatrists. Available online at www.nice.org.uk/nicemedia/live/13629/57542/57542.pdf (accessed 14 June 2013).

This is the NICE guideline that every mental health nurse needs to become familiar with.

Time to Change (2008) *Stigma Shout: Service user and carer experiences of stigma and discrimination.* London: Time to Change. Available online at www.time-to-change.org.uk/sites/default/files/Stigma%20Shout.pdf (accessed 14 June 2013).

This is an excellent report detailing responses from service users and carers about their experience of mental health stigma.

Useful websites

www.nice.org.uk

NICE produces evidence-based practice guidelines for health and social care services in England. All best practice guidelines for mental health practice can be accessed via this site.

www.nmc-uk.org

The Nursing and Midwifery website.

www.rcpsych.ac.uk

The Royal College of Psychiatrists website – very useful for psycho-education literature and reports.

www.time-to-change.org.uk

Time for Change is England's biggest programme to challenge mental health stigma and discrimination.

Chapter 3
Building rapport

Peter Bullard and Simon Grist

NMC Standards for Pre-registration Nursing Education

This chapter will address the following competencies:

Domain 2: Communication and interpersonal skills

1. All nurses must build partnerships and therapeutic relationships through safe, effective and non-discriminatory communication. They must take account of individual differences, capabilities and needs.

1.1 **Mental health nurses** must use skills of relationship-building and communication to engage with and support people distressed by hearing voices, experiencing distressing thoughts or experiencing other perceptual problems.

3. All nurses must use the full range of communication methods, including verbal, non-verbal and written, to acquire, interpret and record their knowledge and understanding of people's needs. They must be aware of their own values and beliefs and the impact this may have on their communication with others. They must take account of the many different ways in which people communicate and how these may be influenced by ill health, disability and other factors, and be able to recognise and respond effectively when a person finds it hard to communicate.

5. All nurses must use therapeutic principles to engage, maintain and, where appropriate, disengage from professional caring relationships, and must always respect professional boundaries.

5.1 **Mental health nurses** must use their personal qualities, experiences and interpersonal skills to develop and maintain therapeutic, recovery-focused relationships with people and therapeutic groups. They must be aware of their own mental health, and know when to share aspects of their own life to inspire hope while maintaining professional boundaries.

NMC Essential Skills Clusters

This chapter will address the following ESCs:

Cluster: Care, compassion and communication

1. As partners in the care process, people can trust a newly registered graduate nurse to provide collaborative care based on the highest standards, knowledge and competence.

By entry to the register:

12. Recognises and acts to overcome barriers in developing effective relationships with service users and carers.

13. Initiates, maintains and closes professional relationships with service users and carers.

3. People can trust the newly registered graduate nurse to respect them as individuals and strive to help them to preserve their dignity at all times.

By entry to the register:

4. Acts professionally to ensure that personal judgements, prejudices, values, attitudes and beliefs do not compromise care.

5. People can trust the newly registered graduate nurse to engage with them in a warm, sensitive and compassionate way.

By entry to the register:

8. Listens to, watches for, and responds to verbal and non-verbal cues.

9. Engages with people in the planning and provision of care that recognises personalised needs and provides practical and emotional support.

Chapter aims

By the end of this chapter you should be able to:

- describe the importance of a therapeutic alliance;
- state what factors make this up and identify factors that both hinder and enhance the therapeutic alliance;
- recognise a rupture in this alliance and the possible reasons behind it;
- reflect on your role in the process and why this is an important part of any therapeutic alliance.

Introduction

Psychological and psychosocial interventions delivered by mental health nurses often appear straightforward in text, with a clear rationale supporting them. Why, then, is it not so easy in practice to work with patients experiencing mental health problems? A number of factors influence how you as a mental health nurse are able to see positive change from your interventions. We have already seen (Chapter 2) that the therapeutic alliance is one of the most important elements of any helping intervention (Cahill et al., 2008; Egan, 2010; Luborsky et al., 2002).

The therapeutic alliance has been given a number of definitions in the literature. Some, such as Horvath and Greenberg (1994), discuss the alliance in the context of psychological therapies, while others (e.g. Egan, 2010) make reference to the alliance and its existence across a multitude of helping roles. An appropriate definition (Horvath and Luborsky, 1993, p562) when considering all helping professions is: *The client's positive collaboration with the therapist against the common foe of pain and self-defeating behaviour.*

Before we further explore the therapeutic alliance, work through the first activity.

Activity 3.1   *Reflection*

Based on the definition given above, consider your own experience of having a supportive relationship with an individual. This could be within a placement or a previous role in which you have supported a patient/client. Use the following prompts to better reflect on this experience.

- Why could this contact be classed as a supportive relationship?
- What (if any) strategies did you as a supporting individual employ that made this therapeutic?
- What was the supported individual's perception of your relationship?
- How did this alliance influence the outcome of the support/intervention delivered?

As this activity is based on your own experience, no outline answer is provided.

From the exercise it should become evident that a therapeutic alliance is important whether you are delivering long-term psychological therapy, or simply supporting an individual with a brief intervention. Egan (2010) has suggested the power of any intervention to help an individual overcome his or her problems will be lost if the therapeutic relationship is poor.

We can also observe the benefit of a strong alliance in other professions.

Scenario

Imagine a patient is seeing the GP about her or his fibromyalgia.

If the patient trusts the GP, feels he or she has considered all aspects of the diagnosis and considers the GP to have expertise in the problem, the patient may be more likely to comply with the doctor's prescription. A GP who has not taken the time to understand the patient and instead prescribes medication without much of a dialogue may find the individual is less compliant with treatment.

We can apply this theory to the mental health nurse. Read the case study below and then complete the activity that follows.

Case study

James is a 35-year-old outpatient with a diagnosis of bipolar disorder. He has received hospital treatment and has now been discharged to continue his recovery in the community. James takes a mood stabiliser, which has helped reduce episodes of mania and depression. He now wishes to become more independent and integrate into the community by going into town to do his shopping. James experiences panic attacks when attempting to do this and Hilary, the mental health nurse supporting him, decides exposure therapy would be an effective intervention.

James is introduced to the intervention but, when he expresses his fear of fainting in crowded places, Hilary rejects the claim and states 'Lots of people like you manage in shops, you will be fine.' James is concerned his fears have not been seriously considered. Hilary moves swiftly into building a hierarchy of exposure tasks. James has very little input and the first step to go to the local shop is suggested for him. James is terrified at this thought but agrees as Hilary insists it should be the first step.

At the next contact James states he was unable to go to the shop and had been more anxious since the previous visit. Hilary tells him he needs to be brave and suggests they try the first step again. James was unable to explain why he had not undertaken the first step.

Hilary receives a message after the session that James would prefer to stop treatment at this point.

It is clear from the case study that, as treatment progressed, James became more reluctant to engage. But why?

Activity 3.2   *Critical thinking*

- What do you think Hilary, the mental health nurse, could have done differently here to increase the chance of a positive outcome?
- How did you observe their therapeutic alliance?
- How do you think the patient, James, experienced their therapeutic alliance?

As this activity as based on your own reflection, no outline answer is provided.

What contributes to the therapeutic alliance?

Over the course of this chapter the contributing factors that help mental health nurses to build strong therapeutic alliances with their patients will be discussed at length. Here we consider an overview of the skills required to build a strong alliance, found in Egan (2010) and applied to mental health nurses.

- The nurse should help the patient to fully understand the nurse's techniques, rationale and value in helping the patient reach his or her goal.
- The intervention should be adaptable to the patient's needs without sacrificing professional standards.
- The approach needs to be collaborative with the patient having a say in all decisions.
- Efforts to enhance the relationship should be considered throughout the intervention or risk losing the power to make change.
- The mental health nurse should try to understand the patient from his or her unique perspective, even if the nurse feels the patient needs to be challenged.
- Criticism, blame and rejection must be avoided and instead a curious stance must be adopted.

This list is not exhaustive and requires ongoing practice and reflection from clinical experience to develop these skills. The following sections in this chapter will further break down the components of the therapeutic relationship and provide opportunities to practise developing skills.

Therapeutic use of self

Now that we have a sound understanding of how a therapeutic alliance can influence a patient's journey through care, it is important to understand what impact we as individuals can potentially have on this. We are all different and our differences are the result of many factors: our personalities, our upbringing, our experiences and our beliefs and values. The skill within any therapeutic interaction is to use this to enhance the relationship we have with our patients by better understanding ourselves. This is an area that is considered in depth in a number of therapies and has been extensively written about, with Peplau (1952) being arguably the most well known within the field of nursing. A greater understanding of self cannot be taught within a few pages, but it is a skill that is honed and developed through practice and the use of tools. It is these tools that we are going to consider here and the use of these will allow you as a practitioner to develop a greater understanding of yourself. The main tools that we will consider here are self-practice, reflection and the use of supervision.

Self-practice

Self-practice has been a feature of cognitive therapy for many years (Beck, 1995; Bennett-Levy et al., 2001; Padesky and Greenberger, 1996) and very simply refers to the self-practice of the interventions we ask our patients to undertake. This allows us to both identify potential obstacles that may come up and also be able to empathise with our patients around the use of these interventions. By doing so we improve our therapeutic alliances. While much of the research is focused on CBT, self-practice is a tool that can be used within any therapeutic area.

Activity 3.3 *Reflection*

Consider your current or most recent practice placement and from this identify one or two interventions that would be helpful for you to self-practise. This might be the use of a thought diary to practise recording thoughts, or practising being detained under a section of the Mental Health Act (you may need to ask a colleague or peer to help here, whom you need to go to and ask for leave from). Record your feelings while doing this and what you found difficult and what was easier. This then helps you to understand better what you are asking your patients to do through your own experiences.

As this activity is based on your own experiences, no outline answer is provided.

Reflection

The Oxford English Dictionary defines 'reflection' as:

> *The action of turning back or fixing the thoughts on some subject; meditation, serious consideration. Recollection, remembrance. The process or faculty by which the mind has knowledge of itself and its workings.*

In healthcare, reflection has a distinct purpose of learning from experience, which encourages further learning and development, and maintains good practice by bridging the theory–practice gap. This allows greater understanding of self and encourages practitioners to become competent and responsive. Reflection is a skill that develops with practice but can be helped with the use of reflective models. These models are very individual and practitioners often have their favourite, but some commonly used ones include Kolb (1984), Gibbs (1988), Driscoll (1994) and Johns (1995).

In Gibbs' (1988) model (Figure 3.1), when describing the situation, it is important to just describe facts and not make judgements or form conclusions. When describing feelings the same applies

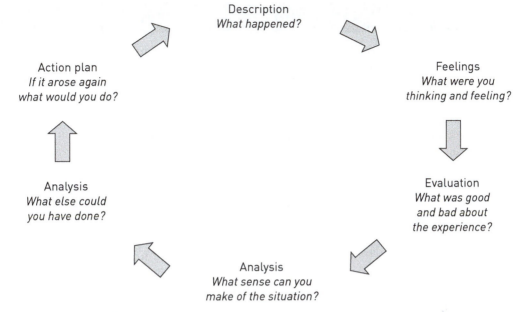

Figure 3.1: Gibbs' (1988) reflective model

here – it should be just feelings, not conclusions. Within the analysis it can also be helpful to explore other people's experience.

The Driscoll model (1994) may seem easier (see Figure 3.2), but can take some practice to fully develop.

'What?' refers to returning to a description of the situation, which can also include feelings. 'So what?' refers to an analysis of the situation, trying to understand the context, again including other people's experience if appropriate. 'Now what?' is aimed at modifying future outcomes and, if necessary, action plans.

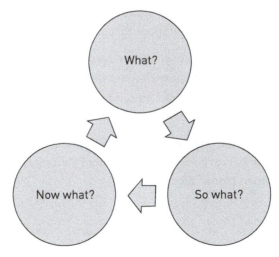

Figure 3.2: Driscoll's (1994) reflective model

Activity 3.4   *Decision making*

Look at the reflective models mentioned above – consult the 'Further reading' list at the end of the chapter for more details – and with a peer/colleague use one to reflect on an experience that you have had recently.

Try the same experience using a different model and compare them with the intention of finding one that meets your personal preference.

As this activity is based on your own experiences, no outline answer is provided.

Supervision

Supervision is a tool that allows us to explore the interactions that we have with our patients. As such it explores our reactions, our patients and our use of interventions and techniques. Much has been written about supervision, but it nonetheless lacks a clear, formal definition (Milne, 2009). Most clinicians describe it as a formal, collaborative relationship with typically a more senior clinician who will have greater clinical knowledge and experience to help the supervisee develop as a practitioner.

Scenario

Neema has just completed a clinical placement, and has been asked to describe her experiences of supervision so far in her clinical placements. She starts to list the components of supervision that she feels would help her to get the most from supervision. She begins by saying how important she feels is the use of a supervision contract that clearly states the expectations for both her and the supervisor.

Neema might also have listed: a collaborative relationship, clear goals, a safe environment, regular time and venue, and clear supervision questions that allow you to develop as a practitioner.

Use this in your next placement to help in your development as a practitioner and understanding of yourself within a clinical context. Supervision can be likened to a muscle: the more you use it the more it develops and becomes more efficient; however, using or stretching it the wrong way can lead to difficulties elsewhere.

Having explored the therapeutic uses of the self, in building rapport, we will now go on to consider the verbal and non-verbal competencies required for a mental health nurse to build and maintain a good-quality therapeutic alliance.

Verbal and non-verbal competencies

Verbal competencies

Active listening skills are integral when engaging in the assessment and treatment phases of an intervention (Myles and Rushforth, 2007). We can break these down into the individual skills that are used to demonstrate listening and understanding, and to help the patient to make sense of her or his problem.

Empathy

The skill of empathy requires the mental health nurse to acknowledge the patient's experience of emotions in relation to the problem discussed. This differs from sympathy, in which the mental health nurse would reply with his or her own perceived experience of the situation. An example of empathy would be the following.

Patient: I feel low, I can't cope, everything is a challenge and I can barely get out of bed. I know I'm letting down my family and friends, and just wish it could all go away.

Empathic response: Things sound really challenging for you.

Sympathetic response: If I was in your shoes I wouldn't be able to get up either. I don't know how you even made it to the appointment today.

Paraphrasing

Paraphrasing demonstrates listening and understanding by restating the key points of what a patient has just said. This skill is useful for managing contact time and can help you make sense of the patient's situation.

Patient: When I go out and the voices talk to me I get really anxious that people are looking at me and think I'm mad. I feel so scared. I have to leave anything I'm doing and get home as soon as possible. It makes getting the day-to-day things done so hard.

Mental health nurse: So you feel anxious and scared when you go out and hear the voices, and this makes day-to-day things difficult?

Reflection

Reflection allows you to acknowledge the difficulty and emotion of a patient's experience. When using reflection you comment on the emotion displayed by the individual. For example, a patient is discussing the impact of her mental health on family life and becomes tearful when mentioning her five-year-old daughter.

Mental health nurse: I noticed when you mentioned your daughter you became tearful.

Summarising

Summarising can be used to help structure a session, display active listening and help the patient make sense of his or her problem. The mental health nurse in this scenario would repeat back to the patient a short summary of the information gathered. This differs from paraphrasing as it is used at the end of sections of information and to review the whole appointment. For example, a patient has just discussed his experience of anxiety in public situations.

Mental health nurse: I'm just going to check I have this right. So when you have to go into busy places such as the supermarket or town centre, you notice your heart beating and feel breathless, hot and sweaty. You feel like people can see you are panicking and that you need to escape, or fear you will pass out. This makes you avoid going to these places as much as possible and leaving quickly if you are in those situations. Have I understood correctly?

The use of these skills should be part of every interaction with a patient and are common factor skills required in any helping relationship (Egan, 2010). Neglect of these skills can damage the mental health nurse's position in the relationship and ability to help the patient in distress.

The next activity allows you to practise each of the above skills with a partner.

Activity 3.5   *Communication*

One person takes the role of the mental health nurse with the other individual to be interviewed. The interviewee can either play the role of a patient, or choose a topic to talk at length about. This should be something he or she feels passionate about, allowing for a display of a range of emotions without feeling uncomfortable. Topics may include:

- experience of health services;
- feelings about medication;
- a difficult work situation;
- a challenging family situation.

The interviewee should start by talking openly about the chosen topic with the mental health nurse using empathy, paraphrasing, reflection and summarising to demonstrate active listening skills. Spend about ten minutes doing this and then consider the following questions.

- What were the benefits of using verbal competencies?
- Did they come naturally to you? If not, which of the skills did you find hardest to use?
- How did this interaction differ from how you would usually communicate with others?
- How did the interviewee experience the interaction?

As this activity is based on your own experience, no outline answer is provided.

Non-verbal competencies

The patient's experience of the mental health nurse is not only based on the nurse's verbal communication but also her or his use of non-verbal listening skills. Myles and Rushforth (2007) suggest the following are important when considering non-verbal characteristics.

Facial expression

You should be aware of your reactions throughout a contact. It is a skill to recognise the patient's responses as well as having an awareness for one's own. There may be long periods when the patient is disclosing information and active non-verbal engagement can be displayed by using subtle nodding, eyebrow expressions and movement of the lips.

Posture

Posture is another individual skill that needs to be developed to make a patient feel comfortable in contacts. Consider how you would usually sit when talking to friends or family. If you naturally cross your arms or legs, or lean away from the individual, this may be something you need to work at in sessions. In a patient contact the mental health nurse should remain upright and open in posture. He or she should lean attentively forward without being intrusive. Try to be aware of any movements made in the session as patients may interpret these differently.

Eye contact

Eye contact should be appropriate at all times. While it is important to maintain eye contact to demonstrate interest, it can also be intimidating if this is held for long periods of time. The mental health nurse should be mindful to maintain sustained periods of eye contact, followed by breaks to look at notes, the patient's body language, time, etc.

Chair position

The seating arrangements should be planned beforehand. Try to remove physical barriers between you and the patient, for example computer desks or tables. While a patient may expect this in a consultation with a doctor, it is not conducive to creating a therapeutic environment. Chairs should be slightly diagonally offset to one another. The mental health nurse and patient should be close enough to share written information, without being intrusive to personal space.

While the concept of learning new skills can provoke anxiety, we are surrounded with opportunities to learn how patients may respond to body language.

Activity 3.6 *Communication*

When you are next in a situation surrounded by others talking, observe what is happening non-verbally.

- How does the person listening respond to what is being said?
- What messages do you think are being sent to the person speaking?

To apply this to yourself, next time you speak with a friend or colleague be mindful of your use of non-verbal communication.

- What happens when you use facial expressions?
- Does your posture change the individual's dialogue?
- If you were to neglect eye contact, how would that impact your conversation?

As this activity is based on your own observations, no outline answer is provided.

Engaging your client

So far we have discussed the therapeutic alliance, its components and how we can remain mindful of its influence throughout assessment and treatment. A key ingredient in enhancing the quality of the alliance, previously highlighted, was the patient's ability to understand how the mental health nurse's interventions may work for him or her (Egan, 2010). Collaboration is required here (Cahill et al., 2008) to ensure understanding and a shared direction for ongoing treatment.

Summarising the session

To ensure patients feel understood it is important that you summarise the information discussed during the initial contact. Egan (2010) states that perceived understanding of the individual's problem should always be clarified to enhance the alliance and demonstrate collaboration. Making assumptions and judgements at this stage could contribute to ruptures in the relationship (see page 59).

This shared understanding allows the mental health nurse to progress the contact to a recovery-oriented approach. The patient can be asked what he or she would perceive as a successful outcome from treatment, leading to more specific goal setting to guide treatment.

Goal setting

A core skill utilised by many clinicians in nursing and therapeutic roles is goal setting. Cahill et al. (2008) suggest the problem discussed at assessment is not a contributor to engagement, but early identification of goals and collaboration over the treatment plan to attain these can enhance the relationship and lead to better outcomes.

The term SMART often goes hand in hand when one thinks of goal setting in helping roles. This allows the patient to begin considering tangible behavioural changes that may improve her or his circumstances.

Concept summary: SMART goals

Specific: Many patients will simply state they wish to feel better. While in a distressed state this is understandable, so the mental health nurse needs to guide the individual to think more specifically about his or her goals. Some useful questions can include asking the patient 'What would you be doing differently if things were to improve?' or 'What would I observe differently about you if you could make changes?' A general wish to 'feel less anxious about social situations' can skilfully be reconsidered as 'going to shops that I currently avoid'.

Measurable: To ensure goals have been achieved they need to be measured. The previous example of 'going to the shops I currently avoid', while specific, lacks measurement as we do not have any indication of how often that would be in recovery. It could mean twice a year. Asking the individual how often he or she would be undertaking the task adds a numeric target to the goal. This also adds a scale to reflect on when later considering the progress of treatment.

Attainable: This needs to be considered in light of the individual supported. It is unlikely that a patient with long-term agoraphobia is going to feel confident enough to travel around the world in two months. The mental health nurse could discuss the patient's history, then look at what could be achieved in two months. Perhaps a more attainable target would be to walk to a local friend's house alone and spend some time talking over coffee once per week.

Resources: Does the individual have the resources to meet her or his goal? Consider a patient with a history of schizophrenia who has experienced multiple difficulties with holding down employment, consequently leading to low income. As part of the patient's recovery he or she may wish to attend a local fitness centre several times per week, but finances may obstruct the patient from doing this. Helping the individual in this case to reconsider her or his goal may lead to using a home exercise plan, jogging and joining a local health promotion scheme, to overcome the issue of poor finances.

Time: Most of us have made a promise to ourselves to change something in our lives for the better. Often things get put off if there is no time limit and other issues get in the way. This should be considered with patients. Setting a time for completion of goals encourages individuals to take small steps towards achieving them. For example, a patient experiencing panic attacks may only challenge his or her anxiety in busy places once a fortnight, if there is no pressure of time to meet the goal. Agreeing a time to review goal outcomes can help motivate and engage patients to interact with set tasks more regularly.

| Activity 3.7 | Critical thinking |

Consider the following three people and write a SMART goal for each. Take into consideration the five steps to developing a good SMART goal with patients.

- Maria struggles to leave the house and get her shopping without the support of her mother. She has always suffered with anxiety about public places but now wants to develop independence so she can find work and develop a social life. She has a few friends in the local area who are supportive.
- Raj has a history of bipolar disorder and in his dysthymic state has gradually withdrawn from those around him over time. His condition is controlled by medication but the damage to his long-term mental health has left him struggling to manage his home surroundings, maintain his well-being and speak to his family.
- Eva has a diagnosis of borderline personality disorder. She becomes highly distressed in her work life and relationships, and when trying to manage finances and utilities. She self-medicates by drinking alcohol excessively seven days per week (120 units per week in total). She realises this is excessive but struggles to manage the multiple demands in her life.

An outline answer is provided at the end of the chapter.

Treatment discussion

Following the development of SMART goals you as the mental health nurse can start to consider treatment options. The inclusion of the patient in treatment planning is likely to result in greater engagement from the individual. Treatment options will differ depending on workplace setting, the skill and background of the mental health nurse and the involvement of other professionals. You will also consider the individual's risk level when agreeing on forward steps. Some examples of treatment may include brief therapeutic intervention or medication management approaches.

Ending the session and next steps

While a collaborative session may end with a sense that all has been covered and the future for treatment is clear, the patient's understanding of next steps should always be clarified (Myles and Rushforth, 2007). Asking the patient 'Can I just check your understanding of what we have agreed?' or 'Just for my own clarity can you tell me your understanding of our treatment plan?' can be helpful ways of eliciting this information. This also offers an opportunity to recap or explain anything the patient is not clear about.

The following session can begin by checking the patient's ongoing understanding of the agreed treatment plan, any tasks he or she was required to complete between the session and his or her experience of completing these. Eliciting this information can create opportunities to problem solve barriers to undertaking the treatment plan. This continued collaboration enhances the therapeutic alliance (Cahill et al., 2008) and can improve patient engagement as he or she is actively involved at each session.

The mental health nurse should remain mindful of the skills required to engage individuals in treatment throughout contacts. Greater engagement can be achieved by ongoing inclusion and ensuring there is a shared vision for treatment and recovery.

Signs of rupture in the relationship

Now that we have a greater understanding of the therapeutic alliance or relationship and how to use skills and techniques to both engage and maintain the therapeutic intervention, we need to understand how some patients may disengage. Disengagement or ruptures in the therapeutic alliance can come about for many different reasons and can be both overt and subtle, and broadly fall into two categories: non-verbal signs and behavioural signs.

Activity 3.8   *Reflection*

Reflect on ruptures you have observed while on placement or signs that you feel are predictive of a potential rupture in the relationship with a patient.

Compare what your reflections suggest with those of your colleagues to see if there are any common themes across placements and with different groups of patients. Were there similarities or themes?

An outline answer is provided at the end of the chapter.

The reasons why ruptures appear in relationships can be many and varied but there are five common problems.

The first concerns the relationship; this may be the relationship that you have with your patient, or could be external to your relationship and may come from relationships that your patient has with family and friends that are influencing his or her interaction with you. These most commonly arise as a result of one individual being driven by his or her own needs. An example of this could be the patient who attends the CMHT as a result of his parents telling him that he needs to seek help, but he does not believe that the CMHT is the right place for him. Or a student nurse who needs to complete a certain intervention with a patient in order for her assessment of practice document to be signed off.

The second problem may be the nature of the illness or condition, such as a psychotic episode or a delusion. The rupture may therefore only be transitory; however, the impact on the patient may also influence the relationship and cause a rupture. An example could be the community nurse who requests a Mental Health Act assessment on his patient, but the patient does not agree with this and continues to harbour distrust towards the worker as a result.

Rupture can also be treatment or intervention driven, where the patient does not see the benefit of the intervention or treatment that has been suggested or applied. An example of this is demonstrated in the case study of Stuart.

> ## Case study
>
> *Stuart had been attending appointments with his CBT nurse practitioner for a number of weeks, having overcome his initial reluctance to engage in CBT due to a relationship clash with his previous worker. This particular session was aimed at helping Stuart to understand how often people have negative views about their physical shapes and the impact that this has on their self-esteem. The practitioner had already decided that the best way to demonstrate this was to ask Stuart to conduct a survey among friends and family about how often, or how frequently, they think about their size or shape. Stuart started to show non-verbal signs of disengagement when this was discussed; he reduced his eye contact and shifted uncomfortably in his seat. This was not picked up by the practitioner who, convinced this was a good idea, continued to discuss how the survey would best be carried out. Stuart felt increasingly uncomfortable with these suggestions and stood up, telling the practitioner that he had to leave.*

A fourth problem is a lack of understanding of either the patient's presenting or current problems or a lack of understanding about how to carry out the task as suggested by the care team. Clearly not understanding the nature and depth of the patient's problem will not allow treatment to be focused and will often leave the patient feeling not listened to. Conversely, if the practitioner does not fully explain the intervention, or the patient does not ask for clarification, the chances are high that she or he will either not carry out the intervention or will disengage from the therapeutic process.

> ## Scenario
>
> *Imagine a situation where the nurse, Patrick, explains to his patient that this particular medication must be taken every day and ideally with food. The patient, Molly, takes the medication, but has always struggled to eat regular meals, and begins to feel sick shortly after taking the medication without food, but continues to take it every day, as instructed. After a few days of feeling really sick Molly stops the medication and avoids the next appointment with Patrick for fear of being readmitted to hospital. Had Patrick explained that the medication is best taken with food as it can cause nausea, and even a glass of milk or a couple of biscuits can stop this nausea, Molly would have continued taking the medication.*

Lastly, transference issues and historical past may also impact negatively on the therapeutic alliance. Transfer is the impact that past interactions have on current relationships and generally relates to feelings that are generated in these interactions. An example of this could be the patient who was verbally and emotionally abused at school by one of the teachers and responds to the practitioner in a timid way due to transference around those in positions of power.

Attending to the ruptures

Attending to a potential or actual rupture within the therapeutic relationship can be viewed either negatively or positively. A negative response from a practitioner would suggest that he or she considered the problem to lie solely with the patient and therefore there would not be anything the practitioner could do to improve the situation. A positive view would be that the practitioner is concerned about this rupture and wishes to learn more to enable this impasse to be overcome.

Activity 3.9   *Reflection*

With a colleague role play a situation in which one of you plays the patient and the other the practitioner. An example of a situation could be a patient who does not wish to take her or his medication.

- The practitioner should first of all take the stance of not wishing to attend to any potential rupture and should insist that the medication has to be taken. Explore how this felt as both patient and practitioner.
- Then the practitioner should take a stance of enquiry, trying to understand the reasons why the patient does not wish to take the medication. Again explore how this felt as both practitioner and patient.

As this activity is based on your own actions, no outline answer is provided.

As you will have gathered from the exercise, the rigid stance taken in the first instance is unlikely to have led to any change in the patient's behaviour without resorting to other means such as use of the Mental Health Act. In therapy a rupture is often viewed as an opportunity to learn, for both the practitioner and the patient, no matter how hard this may feel, and all current intervention work is suspended until the rupture is better understood and managed (Westbrook et al., 2011). What follows are some ideas about how to attend to the ruptures that are taken from a number of therapeutic approaches. Clearly as practitioners you will need to evaluate how useful these may be in a particular situation as there is no 'one size fits all' approach to attending to ruptures; however, as you become more experienced, your skills at both noticing and attending to the ruptures will increase.

Understand the issue better

The first step has to be to fully understand the issue in as non-judgemental way as possible. This generally would utilise the common factors, as described earlier in the chapter, to help re-establish the therapeutic alliance. One of the key aspects of this is to demonstrate empathy:

The state of empathy, or being empathic, is to perceive the internal frame of reference of another with accuracy and with the emotional components and meanings which pertain thereto as if one were the person, but without ever losing the 'as if' condition. Thus it means to sense the hurt or the pleasure of another as he [sic] senses it and to perceive the causes thereof as he perceives them, but without ever losing

the recognition that it is as if I were hurt or pleased and so forth. If this 'as if' quality is lost, then the state is one of identification.
(Rogers, 1959, pp210–11)

Another important aspect of understanding the issue better alongside common factors and empathy is that of using the patient's own language in a way that generates a feeling of understanding between the practitioner and patient. Caution should be exercised here that the language used should be related to the rupture specifically and does not include offensive or inciting language.

Evaluate collaboratively

Once the issue is more thoroughly understood, it can be evaluated in a collaborative spirit. The practitioner should help evaluate the issue using a selection of strategies. For example, treatment goals could be reviewed to see if they are still true for the patient. The stages of change model (Prochaska and DiClemente, 1983) can be helpful to ensure that the practitioner and patient are aligned with regard to treatment or motivation. Alternatively, an advantages and disadvantages list could be constructed that allows both practitioner and patient to explore possible benefits and barriers. The key here is to start to explore the problem with regard to formulating a way to move forward.

Use reflection

The use of reflection and reflective practices will help manage the situation. Supervision, for example, should be a safe place to bring ruptures to discuss and explore and the use of self-practice and self-reflection (Bennett-Levy et al., 2001) can be useful to gain an understanding and empathy for the patient. In CBT practitioners are encouraged to work on their own issues, and in this way they generate both empathy and understanding (Padesky and Greenberger, 1996).

Move forwards

Moving forwards is the final element of dealing with the rupture and this again should be as collaborative as possible. Where possible choices should be offered rather than a fixed approach, as in this way the patient feels more part of the solution, especially if she or he is able to generate some of the options. As practitioners we should always be hopeful of change for the better for our patients, as without this they are also unlikely to believe that positive change can happen.

Some final thoughts with regard to managing the ruptures: it can, if deemed therapeutic by the care team, be useful to involve significant others within the treatment process to aid both understanding and support, although caution should always be practised here and the situation should be fully risk assessed. We, as practitioners, should also not assume that the problem lies with the patient; as we saw earlier with 'Stuart' it was the practitioner's desire to push the intervention that led to the rupture. Conversely, we must be aware that we are there to provide care, we are not friends, although we should always try to be friendly. Finally, don't ignore 'the elephant in the room' – if you as a practitioner feel that something is not right, then it probably isn't, and it makes far more sense therapeutically to address this as early as possible to reduce the chance of the situation worsening. Supervision can be a key element here to help you recognise and manage a potential situation.

> ## Chapter summary
>
> In this chapter we have explored the components of a therapeutic alliance, and examined some of the tools that can be helpful in guiding us to ensure our alliances with our patients are as strong as they can be. We have looked at verbal and non-verbal skills that will aid you in building and maintaining these skills alongside practical interventions that will engage your patients in the process. Like any skill, these need to be practised regularly in your day-to-day interactions with patients and there are some tools used in this chapter that will be helpful for you to explore the therapeutic alliance you have with your patients. We have also considered what a rupture in the therapeutic relationship may look like and explored some of the possible reasons as to why this might have happened.

Activities: brief outline answers

Activity 3.7: Critical thinking (page 58)

Possible goals for these three patients are:

- For Maria: to go to the local shop and my friend's house by myself once per week, by the end of two months.
- For Raj: to build motivation to spend one day per week on housework, shower three days per week and go to my parent's house twice a month, by the end of August.
- For Eva: to reduce alcohol consumption to 60 units per week, with one alcohol-free day, and contact a debt support service to make a budget plan, by the end of two months.

Activity 3.8: Reflection (page 59)

Typical themes or examples are discomfort, anger, expressing cynicism, not completing activities and missing appointments, to name a few.

Further reading

Driscoll, J (1994) Reflective practice for practise. *Senior Nurse*, 13: 47–50.

Gibbs, G (1988) *Learning by Doing: A guide to teaching and learning methods*. Oxford: Oxford Polytechnic.

Johns, C (1995) The value of reflective practice for nursing. *Journal of Clinical Nursing*, 4: 23–30.

Kolb, D (1984) *Experimental Learning*. Englewood Cliffs, NJ: Prentice Hall.

These four works describe the most important models for reflection, which are models you should be familiar with. Reflection in practice is a most important skill.

Useful websites

www.iapt.nhs.uk

Here you will find the Improving Access to Psychological Therapies website, which has information about the programme that supports the implementation of the NICE guidelines for people suffering from depression and anxiety disorders.

www.mind.org.uk

Here you will find information on various aspects of mental healthcare, including CBT, with a more service user-led perspective.

www.rcn.org.uk/development/learning/learningzone

Here you will find online continuing professional development (CPD) resources relating to nursing care, career development and workplace issues. There are pages relating to clinical supervision and reflective practice.

Chapter 4
Questioning skills

Janine Ward

NMC Essential Skills Clusters

This chapter will address the following ESCs:

Cluster: Care, compassion and communication

1. As partners in the care process, people can trust a newly registered graduate nurse to provide collaborative care based on the highest standards, knowledge and competence.

By the first progression point:

5. Is able to engage with people and build caring professional relationships.

2. People can trust the newly registered graduate nurse to engage in person centred care empowering people to make choices about how their needs are met when they are unable to meet them for themselves.

By the first progression point:

1. Takes a person-centred, personalised approach to care.

By the second progression point:

2. Actively empowers people to be involved in the assessment and care planning process.

6. People can trust the newly registered graduate nurse to engage therapeutically and actively listen to their needs and concerns, responding using skills that are helpful, providing information that is clear, accurate, meaningful and free from jargon.

By the first progression point:

1. Communicates effectively both orally and in writing, so that the meaning is always clear.
3. Always seeks to confirm understanding.
4. Responds in a way that confirms what a person is communicating.

By the second progression point:

6. Uses strategies to enhance communication and remove barriers to effective communication minimising risk to people from lack of or poor communication.

Chapter aims

By the end of this chapter you should be able to:

- use a range of questioning styles to communicate with patients;
- reflect, paraphrase, clarify and summarise;
- gather appropriate and relevant information in a timely manner.

Introduction

Case study

Sally has been detained under Section 3 of the Mental Health Act and brought by the police to the Intensive Care Unit where you are working. You have been asked to assess Sally's current mental state. Sally is talking at a very quick rate and jumps from subject to subject; she finds it difficult to understand why she is in hospital. Sally's body language is tense and agitated.

This chapter will focus on introducing a simple questioning technique that will enable you to work through the most difficult of interactions with your patients, including patients like Sally. This will include practical exercises to test your skills and illustrations in the form of case studies and scenarios. First we look at why it is important to learn questioning skills as a mental health nurse. We will then move on to an outline of the types of questions that are useful in patient-centred interviewing. Next we look at the different verbal cues that indicate listening and ensure understanding. We discuss using these questions during risk assessment and, finally, using questioning techniques over different forms of delivering therapy.

Why questioning skills are important

You need to use the technique of questioning in order to make your interviews and assessments patient-centred (Shattell et al., 2007). Good interactions with patients help build an effective therapeutic relationship and help the empowerment of the patient (Egan 2013; Mead and Bower, 2002). When questioning patients, you are not just getting information, in the style of a market researcher in the street. You are building a relationship, which is more important than filling in the spaces on a form.

It is known that dogmatic interview styles, where questions are asked from a list and do not change despite the answers given by the patient, are unhelpful in gaining accurate information. They are often a series of closed questions (Bennett-Levy, 2006), whereas using open and closed questions together can gather a significant amount of useful and relevant information (Richards and Whyte, 2011), and at the same time help build rapport between you. This brings us to the first step of questioning skills: the different types of questions.

Closed questions

A closed question has a closed answer, which leads nowhere. An example is 'Do you hear voices in your head?' This lets the patient say yes or no, but does not encourage her or him to respond with much more information. Other examples of closed questioning are 'Do you take your medication in the morning or evening?', 'What time do you go to sleep', etc. They may not be 'yes or no' questions but they have a limited choice of, or closed, answers. These are good questions when you need *quantitative* information quickly and succinctly, but will elicit very little *qualitative* information.

Activity 4.1   *Critical thinking*

Think about the following questions, and make notes in answer. This will help you think critically about closed questions.

- What mental health situations may benefit from closed question styles?
- In what situations may it not be beneficial to use closed questions?
- What opportunities arise from using closed questioning techniques?
- What threats may arise from using closed questions?
- How might closed questions help in the assessment of Sally?

An outline answer is provided at the end of the chapter.

General open questions

These questions give lots of different opportunities for answering. For example, 'Tell me about your problems' and 'Tell me about your health.' They refer to general issues (e.g. 'health' rather than 'blood pressure') and often appear at the beginning of assessments or patient interviews. They tend to gather a lot of information and encourage a patient to open up about an issue. They allow patients to use their own language. However, it can be almost impossible to get succinct answers or control the direction in which the answers take the conversation.

Open specific questions

These questions tend to be a mixture of closed and open questions, combined to form a semi-open question. They are on a specific subject, but allow the patient to answer at length and in his or her own words, for example 'Tell me more about how this problem is affecting your day-to-day life' or 'What kind of physical symptoms do you get when you are anxious?'

Activity 4.2   *Communication and reflection*

In a group of three or more people, choose one of the questioning styles above to each use in questioning another person within the group. The subject of the questions can be your choice, but for an example, take turns in acting as a famous person. The idea is not to tell anyone who you are but to use the questioning style to find out. You are not able to mix question types.

Reflect on the following questions:

- What did you notice about each questioning style?
- Were any of the styles more helpful than others?

---

continued . . .

- How did you feel using the different styles?
- How do you think the person receiving the questions felt?

Additional activity:

- Try using open general and specific questions in role playing an assessment of Sally: what worked well and what did not?

An outline of example reflections appears at the end of the chapter, but these may vary from your own reflections due to the nature of reflective practice.

You may have noticed that using one particular type of questioning does not really work in gathering useful information. Arguably closed questions will get you the answer you want but will alienate the patient, be very clinician-centred and be unlikely to build a good therapeutic relationship. General open questions may elicit a lot of information but alone cannot provide you with specifics, so you are likely to gather a significant amount of information that is unguided and unspecific. Specific open questions may give you more focused information but you will never get closed answers.

In conclusion, one type of question style alone does not suffice in gathering worthwhile information from a patient. Using all three styles together will enable you to gather more information and in a patient-centred way, a process known as funnelling.

Funnelling

Funnelling is the process whereby a combination of the three styles of question is used to gather information. The idea is that you start with open questions and then focus in on the specific area you need information about, helping the patient open up as you go. Figure 4.1 shows how this can work.

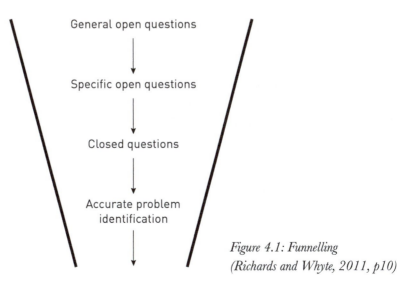

General open questions

↓

Specific open questions

↓

Closed questions

↓

Accurate problem
identification

↓

Figure 4.1: Funnelling
(Richards and Whyte, 2011, p10)

Case study

Sally is interviewed using the technique of funnelling.

A general open question is used to start: 'Tell me about your mental health.'

Then a series of specific open and closed questions is used to gather information on specific topics of interest (see the 'Content of questions' section, page 75).

Sally: *Well, I've been feeling down and depressed all of my life and have dysthymia. But sometimes I get so overinflated that I can't explain it but I feel overwhelming happy and invisible!*

Nurse: *When did you first notice having low mood?* (Specific open)

Sally: *Not sure really, maybe when I was 18?*

Nurse: *OK, so maybe 18?* (Closed)

Sally: *Yes I think so.*

Nurse: *You mentioned dysthymia?* (Closed)

Sally: *Oh yes I did.*

Nurse: *When did you find out you had that?* (Closed)

Sally: *I don't know, I think I saw a psychiatrist once who said I had it.*

Nurse: *Can you tell me more about what mental health help you have had in the past?* (Specific open)

Funnelling questions will lead you to accurate problem identification and enable a patient-centred assessment (Richards and Whyte, 2011). Learning to choose the right type of questions will help you throughout your nursing practice.

Activity 4.3   *Communication and reflection*

Think about which questions may be helpful in the assessment of Sally. Which general open, specific open and closed questions would you use?

- What questions did you think of?
- Which questions do you think will obtain the information you will need to assess Sally effectively?
- How does thinking about using the funnelling techniques in your practice feel?
- Are there any concerns you have about using the technique?
- Is there anything you would do differently next time?
- Is there anything you would do the same next time?

As this activity is based on your own reflection, no outline answer is provided.

Other techniques involved in funnelling

Alongside general open, specific open and closed questions there are several verbal techniques that will help you to understand and correctly identify the main problem. These appear beside the funnel in Figure 4.2.

Although not part of the funnel itself, these four additional skills feed directly into the funnelling process, and it is these skills we will look at now.

Summarising

Summarising, the first of these techniques, will help ensure you have a correct understanding of the patient's problem. It also helps the patient to know you are listening and are processing the information he or she is telling you. Summarising is not repeating the answers given; it is a shortened version, a summary, of what has been said. When you summarise is up to you, but it should ideally fall naturally after a block of funnelling. Here is an example.

Nurse (N): Tell me about your mental health. *(General open)*

Patient (P): I am not very well, I have problems with voices in my head.

N: Tell me more about these voices. *(Specific open)*

P: They happen constantly, there are two of them. Both are people from my past – a teacher and an old GP.

N: How long have you had these for? *(Closed)*

P: At least 15 years, they come and go. They are worse when I am stressed out. Usually I manage to block them out by listening to music.

N: So you have two voices you hear, which has happened for around 15 years. They are a teacher and an old GP. They are worse when you are stressed, but usually you can block them out with music? *(Summarising)*

P: Yes, that's right.

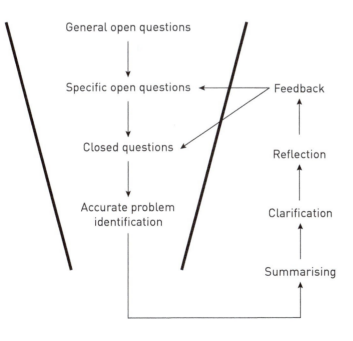

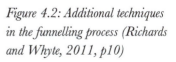

Figure 4.2: Additional techniques in the funnelling process (Richards and Whyte, 2011, p10)

The summary here finishes off a specific funnelled topic, but equally ensures you have understood what has been said, and using intonation to imply a question invites the patient to answer 'yes, that's right' or 'no, you missed something'.

Activity 4.4   *Communication*

Here are three excerpts from clinical interviews. For each one, try summarising what you as practitioner have learned from the patient.

1. *Clinician (C):* Tell me about your main problem.

   Patient (P): I'm depressed and down all the time, I feel so low.

   C: How long has this been going on?

   P: Well at least the last 6 months, but if I think carefully about it, it has been over the last year.

   C: Was there anything that triggered it off last year?

   P: I lost my job as a shop assistant and then I found it difficult to pay bills, my partner is upset with me and I lost a good friend about six months ago.

2. *C:* How is your sleep at the moment?

   P: Well, I'm not sleeping at all.

   C: How much sleep do you think you may be getting?

   P: I don't know really.

   C: OK, well tell me about last night – how did you sleep?

   P: I went to bed about 2200hrs and couldn't get off to sleep; I eventually drifted off about midnight, but I woke up again at 2 and 4am. Eventually I gave in and got up at about 6am.

   C: So what is it that stopped you getting off to sleep?

   P: Well, I was thinking about the day, mulling it over and worrying about the things I had said to others.

   C: Was there anything in particular that happened yesterday?

   P: No, I do this every night; usually I think what a bad person I am and how nothing ever goes right for me.

3. *C:* How is your low mood affecting your day-to-day life at present?

   P: I'm finding it difficult to get out of bed in the morning sometimes; also I find it hard to motivate myself to do anything. I have stopped going out as well.

   C: Do you go out at all?

   P: Yes, I do go to my friend's around the corner occasionally for a coffee, but I haven't been for two weeks now.

   C: How often did you used to go before?

   P: At least twice a week.

   C: What other things do you find difficult to do?

   P: The housework is a real struggle; I know I should do it but I find it difficult to get up and sort it out.

An outline answer is provided at the end of the chapter.

Clarification and reflection

Clarification and reflection are two other key techniques that follow on from summarising. Clarification is gaining clarity or understanding of something the patient has said, for example 'So you sleep six hours in the day?' A clarifying question will typically be a closed question that clarifies points of information and ensures that you have an accurate response.

This is the end of one funnel and will feed into the next set of questioning.

Reflection is stating back to the patient something he or she has just said, to show you understand and are listening. You reflect using the patient's own words, and you can use reflection throughout the dialogue. It invites the patient to clarify what has been said if it is not an accurate reflection. It also gives him or her a chance to correct anything he or she has said.

Let's see how the nurse can use clarification and reflection in the dialogue.

Nurse (N): Tell me about your mental health. *(General open)*

Patient (P): I am not very well; I have problems with voices in my head.

N: Voices in your head. *(Reflection and clarifying)* Tell me more about these voices. *(Specific open)*

P: They happen constantly, there are two of them. Both are people from my past – a teacher and an old GP.

N: A teacher and GP? *(Reflection and clarifying)* How long have you had these for? *(Closed and clarifying)*

P: At least 15 years, they come and go. They are worse when I am stressed out. Usually I manage to block them out by listening to music.

N: So you have two voices in your head, which has happened for around 15 years. They are a teacher and an old GP of yours. They are worse when you are stressed, but usually you can block them out with music? *(Summarising and clarifying)*

P: Yes, that's right.

Feedback

This is the last part of the funnel, and is the information you have gathered so far which fuels the following questions. This depends on what the patient has answered previously and what you need to gather as a professional within your particular setting.

In the example above, the patient hearing voices, the feedback would be further questioning about psychotic symptoms, diagnosis, stressors and other helpful factors.

Scenario

You are assessing Sally, who has come on to the ward with what she describes as dysthymia. Sally has spoken about periods of elation and having had the problem for a number of years. She often jumps from one subject to the next and is difficult to contain. You have been asked to assess Sally's mental health.

continued . . . . •••

Below is an example dialogue of how to assess Sally. The nurse is using the funnelling technique to help her assessment.

Nurse (N): *Hi Sally, can you tell me about your main problem?* (General open)

Sally: *Well I have dysthymia and I just can't stop being low all the time and down all the time and sometimes I feel happy and ecstatic and happy and sad ...*

N (interrupts): *So you have up and downs and feel happy and sad?* (Summarising, reflecting and clarifying with a closed question)

Sally: *Yes, I mean I just cannot control myself. I got picked up by the police because I was chatting to a woman in Superdrug and kept shouting at her about how good I felt and how the world was great and nothing mattered in life ...*

N (interrupts): *OK, so you found yourself unable to be in control?* (Paraphrasing and closed clarifying) *How long have you had this problem for?* (Closed)

Sally: *I don't know really, probably all my life, but maybe a little while. I saw someone once, a head doctor, been in here and there a few times.*

N: *All your life?* (Reflection and clarifying closed)

Sally: *Yes, all my life, it's a terrible shame. I used to be OK when I was at school then something bad happened in the family and I started to find myself doing this! Do you think that woman thinks I am nuts?*

N: *I am sure the woman may have been worried about you and how you are feeling.* (Normalising) *Tell me more about the doctor you saw.* (Open specific)

Sally: *Oh, he was Dr Foster from the Chilterns, it's a mental health hospital in the north. I saw him when I ran away up there, when I was 15 years old.*

N: *So you ran away up north.* (Summarising) *How often have you 'run away'?* (Closed and clarifying)

Sally: *I do it all of the time; I get worried about my life and think it'll be better elsewhere.*

N: *OK, so tell me about what kind of things you have noticed about your mood today.* (Open specific)

Sally: *Well it all started three days ago really, not just today. I started a new relationship with a man from the pub and he told me he would look after me and bought me lots of drinks. I was very drunk. We decided to move in together, that's mad isn't it, but I liked him a lot and had nowhere to stay.*

N (interrupts): *So it started three days ago and you met a nice man you got on with?* (Summarising and clarifying)

Sally: *Yes, he is very nice.*

N: *So why do you have nowhere to stay?* (Closed)

Sally: *Because I ran away from my family up in Hull and found myself here in Southampton with no money or friends.*

N: *OK, so you ran away from Hull. Is there likely to be family looking for you then?* (Closed and clarifying)

Sally: *I suppose there probably is, they are pretty used to me doing this though.*

N: *So they are used to you doing this?* (Reflection and clarifying) *Maybe when you feel a little more relaxed would you be OK with providing me their details?* (Closed)

Sally: *Yes, course, but I can't think right now, my mind is all over the place.*

continued . . .

N: *Sounds difficult for you, what with your mind being all over the place.* (Clarifying and reflective) *Are you on any medication?*

Sally: *Yes, I'm on Tegretol but I haven't had them for a few days as I left them behind.*

N: *OK, so you are on Tegretol, do you know what for?* (Reflection and clarifying)

Sally: *Yes, bipolar I think, that's probably why I'm all over the joint, I just can't think straight, I usually take them in the mornings.*

N: *So you usually take them daily and feel all over the place due to not taking them?* (Clarifying and closed)

Sally: *Yes, I hate the way I am, although I feel very happy today and what do you think, do you think I can go home now? I am feeling much better, how do you think I am?*

N: *So you sound like you're a little up and down in how you feel.* (Closed and clarifying) *Why don't I see whether we can go and find out more about your past treatment and about getting you some medication?* (Closed)

Sally: *OK, yes I feel strange, that might be an idea, I'll wait here.*

In a relatively small space of time the nurse has elicited history, the main problem, potential family and medication, while containing Sally's hyper state.

A question to ask yourself, having read the dialogue, is how you think Sally would feel after this conversation. Try to identify what worked well in the funnelling technique, and ask yourself, how would you feel about interrupting a patient the way the nurse did with Sally?

Content of questions

The next important aspect of questioning skills is the content. The content will depend on your service area. This may be a full mental health assessment, a care planning session or a therapeutic session. Having a brief outline of what is expected of you, for example headings or specific topic areas, can help you to think about your general open questions.

Activity 4.5   *Evidence-based practice and research*

In your placement find out what information you may need to gather in assessments, sessions and other encounters with patients. Based on this information, gather together any pro formas that exist to collate such information, or create your own.

- Think about what questions the topics may generate and the open general questions you may start the topic areas off with.
- Be critical and think about the purpose of each topic area. What is the rationale behind gathering the information and what opportunities does it give you in funnelling information?

As this activity is based on your own practice area, no outline answer is provided.

Using funnelling for the assessment of risk

Assessment of risk is a core skill you will need in your practice. The funnelling questioning technique can help to gather risk information about an individual, both suicidal and regarding risk to and from others. Although there are lots of suggested ways of assessing risk there is no validated or reliable way of predicting suicide (Simon and Hales, 2012). There is often an association with practitioners and patients feeling uncomfortable about asking an individual about risk, which can lead to avoidance on the part of both (Dietrich et al., 2009). However, asking about suicide risk reduces the risk (Aseltine and DeMartino, 2004) and is an important way to understand and assess your patient's problem and provide a suitable care plan for her or his needs.

As you may realise from the nature of general open questions, a risk assessment will not start with a general open question as they are general in nature; therefore questions are always specific when asking about risk. For example, you ask 'Tell me about how you feel?', which is a general open question but is unlikely at any point to gather risk information. Instead you may funnel through the assessment and say: 'Sometimes when people do not feel very well, they have thoughts of being better off dead or of harming themselves – do you have any of these thoughts?' This question aims to normalise asking about the thoughts and is closed, as in assessing risk we would like to know specifics that are as objective as possible. Equally, it may lead on from information you have already gathered from the patient. Here is an example:

Nurse (N): Tell me about your mood. *(Specific open)*
Patient (P): I just feel so hopeless all the time and find myself thinking life is not worth living.
N: So you feel hopeless *(Reflection)* and life is not worth living; tell me more about that. *(Specific open)*
P: Every now and then I think it would just be better if I wasn't here.
N: That must be difficult, to think you would be better off not being here. *(Closed and empathetic)*
P: Yes, suppose it is.
N: How often do you have those thoughts? *(Closed)*

Such lines of questioning can help launch into a risk assessment and start to cover some of the key topics required during the assessment. Using the funnelling techniques to gather information for each specific area can be tunnelled down to specific answers that will help form a thorough picture of the patient's risk.

Activity 4.6   *Evidence-based practice and research*

In your practice area gather information about what topics are covered in the service's risk assessment and look at the local protocols for assessing risk.

- What does the initial risk assessment look like, what questions may you need to ask, and how might you ask these?

---

continued . . .

- Think about the funnelling technique and how the questions may look within your interaction with patients.

As this activity is based on your own practice area, no outline answer is provided.

So which topics may a risk assessment cover? Well there are a lot of suggested questions that may be covered in the research, although risk assessment is not meant to be robotic questioning (Simon and Hales, 2012). Table 4.1 gives some examples of risk to self.

Each of the questions will give you specific information about risk to that patient; however, if you remember the feedback part of the funnel, not every question will need to be asked. This will depend on the patient's answer.

Answers to the questions will give you an understanding of the patient's formulation of risk. This is a summary of what you think the risks are and why. For example:

'Sally is at low risk in the short term as although she has thoughts of ending her life, she has no plans, holds hope for the future and has support from her partner. However, there is potential for Sally's risks to herself to increase as she feels that losing her job, which is likely, may lead her to take an overdose. Sally has done this in the past with the intent to die.'

This paragraph gives a brief overview of the information you gathered and your decision making based on the information you have gained. It is a key competence of a mental health nurse to make thorough risk assessments and make decisions about care (NMC, 2010a).

Thoughts	intent, what are these, how long have they had them, how often do they have them, when are they worse or better?
Past	what has happened, how lethal was it, what led up to it, what was the intent, did they seek support, how many times, what has stopped them?
Actions and plans	do they have any, how specific are these, do they have means, have they researched suicide/self-harm, do they intend acting on these thoughts?
Protective factors	what are they, who are they, why do they stop them, do they see them often or have any problems with protective factors?
Hope	how hopeful or hopeless does the patient feel, what hopes do they hold for the future, do they think they will get better?

Table 4.1: Questions about a patient's risk to self

Case studies

Case 1: Steve

Steve has had thoughts on several days in the last two weeks of being better off dead. He has tried several times in the past to end his life, always by overdosing on pills in the house. This has been over-the-counter medication and has always been an impulsive act. Steve has not had to have any treatment for overdose in the past – he states he just gets into bed and goes to sleep. Steve's intent on his past attempts were to go to sleep and he denies actually wanting to end his life. He has always done this when someone was coming back to the house or he would be found. Steve has no current plans but does have access to over-the-counter medication in his house locked in a cupboard that his wife Sarah keeps the key for. He has no current intent to end his life and feels that there is nothing in particular that would mean he would try to end his life again. This is because, since his last attempt five years ago, Steve and Sarah have had a baby who is now three and Steve cannot and will not end his life because of his son. Steve feels hopeful his life will get better and is accessing help to promote this.

Case 2: Debbie

Debbie has no thoughts to end her life, no plans or no intent. She has harmed herself in the past in her teens by cutting her thighs with a bread knife without requiring hospital attention. She feels very stupid about this and felt she did it for attention and to release pressure she felt when being bullied at school. Debbie has never thought about harming herself since and would not do so as her partner is supporting her and she is in a very loving relationship. Debbie feels she would seek help if things worsened and feels hopeful for the future.

Case 3: Hannah

Hannah has thoughts daily of escaping from her life, but she has no plans for how she might do this and is very clear this is not about ending her life, but more about getting away from it all. Hannah has not tried to end her life in the past and has no current intent to do this now. She has a close family but feels that this is one of the reasons she needs to get away. Hannah feels very hopeless and is not sure where her life may go in the future. She hopes that something bad will happen to her accidentally so that she doesn't have to continue living the current life she has. Hannah would seek support if things did worsen with her mood and knows seeking support is important to her.

Activity 4.7 — *Communication and decision making*

Write a risk formulation for each patient in the case studies above.

An outline answer is provided at the end of the chapter.

Funnelling helps to gather the specific information a practitioner requires in making a thorough assessment of a patient's risk. It is patient-centred and follows on from feedback from other questions asked. Risk formulations can be made and used to summarise the patient's given information.

So now you have learned about funnelling and how it might help your practice, let's come back to Sally and a final exercise.

Activity 4.8   *Communication and reflection*

In a group of three, role-play a mental health assessment with one observer, a patient and a practitioner. The patient is Sally, and the practitioner should use the funnelling techniques described throughout the chapter. Gather information on the main problem and how it is impacting on the patient's day-to-day life. Find out goals of treatment and medication, and assess risk to self.

Reflect on how you felt about asking the questions.

- How did the patient feel?
- What went well?
- What didn't go well?
- How might you use these techniques in practice?

As this activity is based on your own role-play, no outline answer is provided.

Chapter summary

Questioning skills are important to build a therapeutic relationship with your patients and gather the imperative information you require to make a decision about care and treatment.

Funnelling is a particular technique that draws together general open, specific open and closed questions along with summarising, clarification and reflection to produce feedback for the next line of questioning.

Such questioning can give specific information about the patient while being patient-centred and empowering. This line of questioning can help provide a thorough risk assessment and prevents the questions asked being a series of tick boxes or robotic interview styles.

Using funnelling within your nursing practice will be useful in your therapeutic sessions and encounters with patients.

Activities: brief outline answers

Activity 4.1: Critical thinking (page 68)

Beneficial situations for closed question styles may include ICUs in times of crisis, when someone is unable to concentrate on given information and questioning, medication distribution, reading Mental Health Act rights, room searches and security checks, and mental state examinations prior to leave – situations that require specific information that is to the point and quickly established.

Situations where closed questions may not be beneficial include group therapies, care planning, Care Programme Approach (CPA) and ward rounds, therapy or one-on-one sessions, heightened mental health states, and de-escalation situations – situations in which therapeutic relationships need to be built, personalising sessions and those situations requiring more detailed answers.

Opportunities arising from using closed questioning techniques may include clarification of information from patients that is difficult to obtain, or gathering demographic details, which may lead on to further questions, for example what medication a patient is on. This may lead to understanding attitudes to medication and concordance.

Threats from using closed questions may include heightening a situation that requires questioning or statements that are open and therapeutic rather than closed and direct. Patients may feel they have been not listened to or are being directly spoken to without empathy. Threats may include those to the therapeutic relationship.

Closed questions may help Sally in situations where a closed answer is useful. For example, reading Mental Health Act rights and seeking understanding in times of crisis where objective clear answers are needed – i.e. did you cut yourself with this glass? – and when administering medication.

Activity 4.2: Communication and reflection (pages 68–9)

Each questioning style has a purpose but cannot be used alone. Closed questions feel easy to use but are very specific; they feel difficult to pose as you may need to have an idea about what you need to ask the person. You lead the conversation in closed questioning styles. Open questions that are general elicit too much information and may feel like they have no real direction. Often these gather lots of information but used alone it is hard to get specifics. The reliance on this question type is on the patient giving relevant information. Specific open questions are much better at gathering information but again rely on the patient giving relevant information. Each type has its advantages and disadvantages and feel different to both you and the patient. Closed questions can be very powerful and expert, while general open questions can feel undirected and unprofessional; this impacts on the relationship between you and the patient. Specific open questions most probably are beneficial if asked on their own but lack the clarity of closed questions to move the conversation on.

Activity 4.4: Communication (page 72)

Excerpt 1
C: OK, so just to summarise what you have said so far, you have been feeling down for about a year, but really noticed it in the last six months. Losing your job triggered this off and since then you have had problems with paying bills and upsetting your partner. More recently your friend has passed away?

Excerpt 2
C: So to summarise – you think you are getting little sleep, waking up in the night and finding it difficult to get back to sleep. You mull over the day's events and that keeps you awake?

Excerpt 3
C: You are finding it difficult to motivate yourself at times and you haven't been to see your friend for coffee, which you used to do a lot. You're also finding the housework a struggle?

Activity 4.7: Communication and decision making (page 78)

Case 1: Steve
Steve is currently low risk in the short term as, although he has thoughts of being better off dead, he has no plans or intent to end his life and past attempts have always been to go to sleep rather than ending his life. Steve has a child and states he would never do anything to end his life since having his son, therefore he is unlikely to try to end his life unless something were to happen to his son.

Case 2: Debbie
Debbie is low risk in the short term as she has no current thoughts, plans or intent and her hopefulness is high. Debbie's risk in the long term is also low as, although she has harmed herself in the past by cutting,

she feels she would not do this again as her partner supports her and the past attempts were for attention and emotional release.

Case 3: Hannah

Hannah is low risk to herself from suicide and self-harm in the short and the long term as, although she has thoughts, these are of being better off away from her current life situation rather than of hurting herself. She has no plans and intent and, although she is very hopeless about her situation, would not end her life.

Further reading

Burnard, P (1997) *Effective Communication Skills for Health Professionals.* Cheltenham: Chapman and Hall.

This book includes a number of communication skills for health professionals. More can be read on funnelling and counselling skills in Part 2.

Morrisey, J and Callaghan, P (2011) *Communication Skills for Mental Health Nurses: An introduction.* Maidenhead: McGraw Hill.

This book has a comprehensive list of questioning styles and techniques that will help to underpin the funnelling technique outlined within this chapter.

Myles, P and Rushforth, D (2007) *A Complete Guide to Primary Care Mental Health.* London: Robinson.

This is a handbook on all aspects of primary mental healthcare and includes DVD clips of assessments of common mental health problems and of risk assessments. It specifically covers questioning techniques and has a range of exercises to test your skills.

Richards, D and Whyte, R (2011) *Reach Out: National programme student materials to support the delivery of training for psychological wellbeing practitioners delivering low intensity interventions* (3rd edition). London: Rethink.

This includes all of the questioning techniques outlined in the chapter along with the role of psychological well-being practitioners, who use funnelling as a main technique in their assessment of mental health problems.

Useful websites

http://cebmh.warne.ox.ac.uk/csr

This is the Centre for Suicide Research centre based at the University of Oxford; it has numerous papers and resources on assessing suicidal risk and self-harm.

www.iapt.nhs.uk

This site has video clips of assessment using the funnelling technique and how it might look in practice. It supports the *Reach Out* materials (see Richards and Whyte (2011) above).

www.skillsyouneed.com

Under the interpersonal skills section of this site there are brief outlines and examples of interpersonal skills and questioning types.

Chapter 5
When communication becomes challenging

Yvonne Middlewick

NMC Essential Skills Clusters

This chapter will address the following ESCs:

Cluster: Care, compassion and communication

6. People can trust the newly registered graduate nurse to engage therapeutically and actively listen to their needs and concerns, responding using skills that are helpful, providing information that is clear, accurate, meaningful and free from jargon.

By the first progression point:

3. Always seeks to confirm understanding.
4. Responds in a way that confirms what a person is communicating.

By entry to the register:

8. Communicates effectively and sensitively in different settings, using a range of methods and skills.
10. Acts autonomously to reduce and challenge barriers to effective communication and understanding.
12. Uses the skills of active listening, questioning, paraphrasing and reflection to support a therapeutic intervention.

7. People can trust the newly registered graduate nurse to protect and keep as confidential all information relating to them.

By the first progression point:

2. Protects and treats information as confidential except where sharing information is required for the purposes of safeguarding and public protection.

By entry to the register:

6. Recognises the significance of information and acts in relation to who does or does not need to know.
9. Acts within the law when confidential information has to be shared with others.

Chapter aims

By the end of this chapter you should be able to:

- explain what can affect communication and make it more difficult in mental health nursing;
- recognise the effects that cognitive impairment can have on communication;
- reflect on your assumptions, values and beliefs and their impact on how you communicate with others;
- describe different strategies to break down some of the barriers to communication.

Introduction

As we have discussed in the preceding chapters, communication is an essential skill for mental health nurses. Both nurses and patients can have difficulties with communication: for patients this can range from levels of distress caused by their mental health problems to cognitive impairment, which may affect their ability to process information. For the nurse, if you are anxious, frightened or lack confidence this may impact on your ability to communicate effectively or may escalate a potential area of conflict.

The Nursing and Midwifery Council (NMC, 2008, 2010a) emphasises the importance of being able to communicate effectively in order to build therapeutic relationships. Communication has been identified as one of the '6Cs' in the *Compassion in Practice* policy document (Commissioning Board et al., 2012). In fact, excellent communication should underpin everything that you do as a nurse and is fundamental in meeting the challenges of providing the other five elements of the 6Cs: care, compassion, competence, courage and commitment. Therefore, being self-aware and having an understanding of your patient's experiences is vital in developing a caring and compassionate relationship. These skills will also help you when communication becomes more challenging.

This chapter will focus on issues related to cognitive impairment and strategies that can be used to help you reach out and make a connection with your patient. This will help you begin the process of building a therapeutic relationship even in challenging situations. Much of this can be accomplished by gaining an understanding of what it would be like to be in your patient's position. This can be achieved by effectively communicating with your patients and their carers to build relationships to ensure that they are at the centre of their care experience (Mind, 2011; National Collaborating Centre for Mental Health, 2012; NMC, 2010a).

What makes communication challenging or difficult?

There are many things that can affect the ability to communicate with patients and their carers and we will be considering some of these later. What is important is always to consider holistically the person you are caring for. People in distress – whether patients or their carers – can understandably become focused on that distress.

Scenario

Sarah was admitted under Section 2 of the Mental Health Act 1983 (amended 2007) following a serious suicide attempt. During handover to the night staff Sarah was described as being withdrawn, although it had been noted that over the last couple of days she had been frequently asking to leave the ward and at times became angry and aggressive with the staff when she could not leave. Late into the evening, when Sarah was

continued . . .

sitting on her own, Jane, one of the staff nurses, went to chat to her. Sarah was initially not keen to chat so Jane just sat with her for a while and then asked her to tell her a little about herself. Sarah started to tell her about how she had really enjoyed studying art at college and had thought she had met her soulmate while she was there. Even though they were both just 18 years old, they were both thrilled when she found out she was pregnant. Sarah had a late miscarriage and both of them were distraught. The difficulties they had managing their grief and some of the hurtful things people had said, such as 'You are young, there will be plenty of other opportunities', put a strain on her and her partner, which Sarah perceived as leading to the breakdown of their relationship. Sarah was understandably upset when talking about this, and then she disclosed to Jane that it was the anniversary of the loss of her baby the next day and that she just wanted to go down to the river to have some quiet time to think about her baby, but that no one would help her. Jane asked if she had explained this to anyone else, to which Sarah replied that no one had really taken the time to talk to her about anything much since her admission.

As the above scenario demonstrates, there may be many things affecting that person at that moment in time, so it is important that you develop your assessment skills, of which communication is an important part. You need to ensure that you find out any other contributing factors that may be affecting communication, such as people's previous experiences. These may impact on any preconceptions you have of the patient or his or her carer. If you think about always treating people as you would want to be treated yourself, this is a good starting point.

Working as a mental health nurse you will frequently encounter people with altered cognitive processes and it is important to consider how these might impact on communication. By considering such challenges, you can begin to develop strategies to help you maximise your potential for communicating in challenging situations. Developing your skills as a reflective practitioner can help you consider how to use yourself therapeutically. Brown (2012, p20) suggests that *reflective practice is at the heart of a therapeutic use of self* and, although at times this may not be entirely comfortable as we explore our inner processes, it should ultimately be a positive developmental experience that has a positive impact on patient care. The NMC (2010a) has also placed an emphasis on the importance of both reflection and supervision as means of considering the impact of working in mental health on yourself and your practice.

Activity 5.1   *Reflection*

Think about your experiences in practice so far, or if you have not yet cared for patients with mental health problems think about experiences from your life.

Make a list of the sort of things that make communication challenging. Try to think widely and not just about diagnoses related to mental health.

Keep your list and compare it to the discussion below.

An outline answer is also provided at the end of the chapter.

You may have highlighted issues relating to patients and their carers or perhaps the multi-disciplinary team. In this chapter the focus will be on patients and their carers, although you may find that the fundamental principles are transferable to any field of practice. We will start by considering areas of practice that student nurses have reported that they find challenging.

Cognitive impairment

Cognitive impairment is a term you may be familiar with. This term is frequently used to refer to issues patients may be having with their memories. Usually when healthcare professionals are using the term cognitive impairment, they mean *when a person has trouble remembering, learning new things, concentrating, or making decisions that affect their everyday life* (Walker et al., 2013, p1). This is most commonly linked with people with dementia; however, if you take another look at the definition above, in particular having trouble concentrating, then it seems that cognitive impairment can affect anyone. It is not exclusively the realm of people with mental health issues.

> ## Activity 5.2   *Reflection*
>
> Have you ever experienced cognitive impairment? If so, how did this affect your ability to speak to and listen to others? Make a list and keep it for consideration below.

It would be unusual if you had never experienced impaired cognition, which can be caused by a very high temperature (pyrexia), or indeed having drunk too much alcohol. You may also have experienced this type of confusion if you have had medication side effects. If you consider some of the people you have cared for with depression, schizophrenia or bipolar disorder, there may be times when the above definition of cognitive impairment may well seem to apply to them. During a period of crisis there may be a significant impact on a person's ability to make decisions about his or her life, which may continue once the person begins his or her recovery journey.

In mental healthcare recovery does not necessarily mean that the person will be free from mental health problems, but that he or she is able to live a fulfilling life by accepting and overcoming the challenges presented (Deegan 1988; Repper 2012). Although healthcare professionals are only a small part of a person's life and ultimately their recovery, they are often involved at times of crisis. Staff can exhibit behaviours that can either support or inhibit patients starting their recovery journeys (Mind, 2011; National Collaborating Centre for Mental Health, 2012).

> ## Case study
>
> *John, a student nurse, is talking to Lucy about why she had been admitted to the clinical area. He was interested in what she was telling him about her family. He asked her about some therapy she had been involved in earlier in the week and what day it had taken place. Although Lucy could remember the therapy and told John about it, she could not recall which day it had been. She asked John what day it was today and he*

continued . . .

struggled to remember, then told her Wednesday (it was actually Thursday). That prompted her to remember that the therapy took place on Monday. However, later she overheard John reporting to the registered nurse that she was slightly confused.

Activity 5.3   *Critical thinking*

- How do you think Lucy felt when she heard this?
- What do you think might have contributed to Lucy's inability to remember what day it was?
- Have you ever been unable to remember what day it is?

As this activity is based on your own critical thinking, no outline answer is provided.

Lucy was angry and upset that she had been labelled as confused, just for not remembering what day it was. The difficulty was that all the days were pretty much the same for Lucy in the inpatient unit. When she is at home she has a defined structure to her days, which she chooses, so on the whole she is pretty clear what day it is. If the nurse had taken more time to explore the view he had about Lucy being 'confused', he may have realised that due to her current low mood she had not been eating and drinking properly. She had developed urinary frequency, which she was too embarrassed to share and which resulted in a urinary tract infection (UTI). Both Lucy's low mood and the UTI could contribute to appearing 'confused'; however, labelling someone and not properly exploring the situation may be unhelpful and stigmatising as well as a barrier to the person engaging with services (National Collaborating Centre for Mental Health, 2012). Many people have complex lives and people who have mental health issues may have complicated and distressing histories. As a nurse you are well placed to listen with care and compassion to the stories that your patient chooses to share. This should be seen as a privilege, not viewed as a chore in the nurse's busy shift.

There may be times when you cannot remember the day, for example if you are working shifts and have different days off in the week or when you are on holiday. What day it is may be unimportant at different times in your life; the important thing is not to label people as this can undermine their sense of well-being (Kitwood, 1997).

Auditory verbal hallucinations

Many of the patients who come into contact with mental health services may be hearing voices. It is not uncommon for these to be particularly distressing, although some people report that the voices they hear are comforting or that if the voices stop they feel a sense of loss.

When healthcare professionals talk about patients hearing voices they mean that they cannot hear the phenomenon as the patient does. Staff may make this distinction, but it is important to consider the emerging scientific evidence. Functional magnetic resonance imaging (fMRI) and positron emission tomography (PET) scanners provide scientists with images of brain functions.

These techniques have been used to explore the neurobiological experiences of auditory verbal hallucinations. The brain is a complex organ and there is consensus among scientists that areas of the brain are active during the experience of auditory verbal hallucinations, although the exact pathophysiology is yet to be determined (Diederen et al., 2011; van Lutterveld et al., 2013; Vercammen et al., 2011). Although the voices may not be audible to the nurse, the patient's brain is being activated and the physiological impact of this continues to be explored. The impact on a person's life may be more apparent and it is the role of the mental health nurse to support patients in managing this.

Activity 5.4   *Critical thinking*

Spend 30 minutes or so listening to some music you enjoy through earphones. Turn the volume to a level where it is comfortable and try having a conversation with someone you know; do not turn your music down. Make a note of how easy or challenging this is.

Now spend 30 minutes listening to some music that you are not so keen on, ensuring that it is at a similar volume to the music you enjoyed, and again have a conversation and make notes as above.

Once you have done this consider the following questions.

- Was having a conversation possible?
- Was it easier or more difficult with the music you did not enjoy?
- What strategies did you use to enable a conversation to take place?
- Did the person you were having the conversation with do anything differently?

As this activity is based on your own observations, no outline answer is provided.

This is a very simplistic way of simulating the experience of hearing voices; however, when you are listening to music through earphones you will be stimulating the hearing pathways of your brain in a similar way to people who have auditory verbal hallucinations. This part of their brains is already occupied so, as you can imagine, it means that they may find listening to you more challenging. Think about some of the strategies you used to hold a conversation. Perhaps you had to really concentrate on what the other person was saying or ask them to repeat themselves several times. You may have spoken quite loudly in response, not with the intention of being aggressive but just so that you could hear yourself above the music. Perhaps you came across as being more irritable when having a conversation while listening to music you did not like, or maybe you were unaffected for 30 minutes. Imagine if the less desirable noise was with you all the time. This may impact on your overall behaviour and thus how you are viewed by the people around you.

If the person having the conversation with you could not see that you were listening to your iPod, he or she may have judged you as distracted or just not listening, without fully understanding why this might be the case. Some patients find that the auditory hallucinations have a calming effect and they may be distressed by the fact that healthcare professionals are trying to stop them, usually with medication. Other patients may find them extremely distressing, and it is usually this group of people who come into contact with healthcare services when the hallucinations having a negative impact on their lives.

For additional information on the experiences of hearing voices you should consider first-person accounts. The Hearing Voices Network (www.hearing-voices.org) contains recent experiences of people and will give you insight into the differing experiences that people have.

Staff: a barrier to communication?

You may have noticed in some of the discussions above that the interactions between patients, carers and staff can be therapeutic by providing a supportive environment. There are also times when you may notice that staff can create a barrier to communication or indeed escalate an already difficult situation. If you reconsider the impact of the behaviour of the staff in the case study related to Activity 5.3, you might be able to clearly see the potential triggers caused by the staff that are likely to escalate a situation; you may also want to consider this when you get to Activity 5.8. NICE (2005) recognised that it is important that staff receive training in managing escalating situations and, in particular, are aware of the impact of their verbal and non-verbal behaviour. To understand when a situation is escalating you need to spend time getting to know people so that you can recognise subtle changes in behaviour that enable you to be proactive in addressing issues early. Once you recognise that there is an issue you need to actively manage it. If you are unsure about what to do, or you begin to feel uncomfortable in the situation, you should use these feelings as a trigger to seek support from more experienced members of staff.

Whenever you are in a situation where communicating with your patient is challenging, consider how you are reacting and whether you are making it more or less challenging. Being able to reflect on these situations and discuss them with someone more experienced, such as your mentor, will help you to develop your skills.

If you feel frightened or are made angry by someone's behaviour, it is likely to show in your verbal and non-verbal body language. You may find yourself speaking more loudly or more quickly, which, rather than making yourself heard, may make the person you are interacting with more agitated, angry, aggressive or frightened. Try to imagine being in the other person's shoes at that moment, as this can help you consider what you might be able to do to help. If you apply the core values of the '6Cs'– care, compassion, competence, communication, courage and commitment (Commissioning Board et al., 2012) – this should help you consider if your approach is appropriate.

Being a reflective practitioner was touched on earlier in this chapter. As a nurse, you need to be able to explore situations such as those where communication becomes challenging by being open and honest with yourself about the part you played. This is important in developing as a skilled practitioner. It is not possible to prepare for all the situations that you will experience as a mental health nurse, but what you need to do is build up your toolkit so that, when a tried and tested strategy does not work, you can delve into your toolkit and try something different. Sometimes people behave in unexpected ways, so being able to reflect on your contributions, reactions and behaviours will help you to become a better practitioner throughout your career.

Strategies to help communication

The art and science of nursing

There has been much debate over the years about the art and science of nursing. The 'art' is often described as the development of caring relationships between the nurse and the patient, and the 'science' aspect is evidence-based practice (Castledine, 2010; Norman, 2009). This is particularly poignant in mental health nursing where patients are reliant on the interpersonal skills of nurses to support them in times of stress.

While the art of nursing is important, it is also extremely important that you don't neglect the science side of your knowledge base. If you consider what has been said above about nursing as an art and a science, it is impossible to see how nurses can practise without both elements. There are many things that are not yet understood about mental illness and how some of the treatments given actually work, two examples of which are electroconvulsive therapy (ECT) and lithium. As discussed above, relatively recent techniques for brain imaging are helping science to gain an understanding of the processes involved. If you neglect your understanding in these areas, it is easier to label someone with auditory verbal hallucinations as 'being difficult' rather than treating her or him compassionately, or someone with a diagnosis of dementia as having 'challenging behaviour' rather than a degenerative brain disease for which, currently, there is no cure. Lack of curiosity about your patients may prevent you from truly understanding their experience of ill health and the impact that it has on their lives. This in turn may prevent you from escorting them on their recovery journeys during the times you are needed. You need to develop your skills in the art of building therapeutic relationships as well as being up to date with the evidence base for your practice. Becoming a reflective practitioner can also help you to consider both of these aspects of your nursing practice.

Treating people in a respectful, compassionate way while ensuring that you view them as equals and never 'give up' on them is important to users of mental health services (Middlewick, 2013). Repper (2012, p109) says the literature reveals three factors that are important in helping people on their recovery journey: *hope and hope-inspiring relationships, taking back control over your life, opportunity and participation.*

There has been work done within the field of dementia care that has considered the 'importance of being a person' and what it might mean to undermine this position. If you explore what is being offered in this area of research it does not take much imagination to consider how helpful this may be in other areas of practice.

Activity 5.5 _Reflection_

Make a list of things you do that make you feel good about yourself. This might include things that you do for yourself, such as having your hair cut regularly, or the relationships you have with others, such as meeting with your best friend once a month.

---

continued . . .

At the other end of the spectrum make a list of things that make you feel less good about yourself; again consider this from the perspective of things you might do and your relationships/interactions with others.

Keep your list and consider your answers in light of the discussion below.

An outline answer is also provided at the end of the chapter.

Promoting well-being

Kitwood (1997) discusses at length the importance of understanding the person behind the illness. He founded the Bradford Dementia Group, which continues its research into improving the experiences of people with a diagnosis of dementia. Although you may be thinking that you are not planning to work with older adults and that Kitwood's work appears dated, there are many transferable skills that can be acquired by understanding the principles he promotes.

In Activity 5.5 you were asked to consider things that make you feel good and less good about yourself. These elements may play an important part in contributing to you as a person and therefore your sense of well-being. Not attending to key aspects on your list that make you feel good, or finding that more of the things that make you feel less good keep happening, may impact on your feeling of well-being and undermine personhood. Kitwood (1997, p8) describes personhood as *a standing or status that is bestowed upon one human being by others, in the context of relationship and social being.*

Kitwood (1997, p8) goes on to state that personhood *implies recognition, respect and trust.* Although he may be referring to this from the context of dementia care, there are clear parallels with recovery-focused care and promoting health and social inclusion (Aslan and Smith, 2012; National Collaborating Centre for Mental Health, 2012; Repper, 2012). For patients to be able to identify what they need to do to keep themselves well may be the first step in the process of self-management. Being able to recognise when they are not doing the things that usually keep them well may enable people to put in interventions early so that they can maintain their sense of well-being, for example ensuring that they eat regularly when they may not feel like eating or making themselves visit friends when they may feel like isolating themselves. Equally, understanding when personhood is undermined, or identifying triggers, which may lead to a deterioration in mental health, is another step towards self-management. Being aware of these factors may lead to timely interventions that may enable a person or his or her family to have minimal contact with mental health services.

While the above discussion is centred around the recognition of what a person may do to maintain a sense of well-being, Kitwood (1997, pp46–7) identified 17 ways in which other people may undermine a patient's personhood; these include treachery, disempowerment, infantalisation, intimidation, labelling, stigmatisation, outpacing, invalidation, objectification, ignoring, imposition, withholding, accusation, disruption, mockery and disparagement. He calls these acts that undermine well-being *malignant social psychology.*

Activity 5.6   *Critical thinking*

- Gain a copy of Tom Kitwood's book *Dementia Reconsidered* or access the document by De Bellis et al. (2009) through the following website: http://nursing.flinders.edu.au/comeintomyworld, or search the internet for an overview of Kitwood's 17 elements of malignant social psychology.

- Read the descriptions of malignant social psychology given, then consider these within your own practice. Try to think about them within the context of the different groups that you have been working with.

- Make a note of any that you have seen done or have done yourself. Do any of these link with the list you made above regarding things that make you feel less good? If any of these were done to you, how would they make you feel?

As this activity is based on your own observations, no outline answer is provided.

It is likely that having any of these done to you would probably make you feel at the very least not particularly good and, at the other end of the spectrum, perhaps you would feel angry. At the beginning of the chapter we met Sarah who was labelled by the day staff as 'angry' and 'aggressive'. However, once Jane took the time to talk to Sarah it became apparent why she was so keen to leave the clinical area. Perhaps if the staff had taken the time earlier to try to explore the situation, they may have been able to prevent her feeling so angry by understanding her motivation for wanting to leave and facilitating an alternative to enable Sarah's needs to be met.

When communication becomes challenging it is important to be even more self-aware so that you don't unintentionally undermine a person's sense of well-being. If you do, it is important that you recognise this early enough to apologise and prevent the likelihood of a situation escalating. Once a person begins to feel angry or irritated, it becomes more challenging to reverse the situation. It is also possible that you may not be the person who caused the situation, but that everything now feels like it is being directed at you. Being able to demonstrate that you are interested in helping the person by listening to him or her, with the intention of trying to help, can support the person.

Emotional intelligence

Emotional intelligence is considered to be an important part of the development of a mental health nurse (Freshwater and Stickley, 2004; van Dusseldorp et al., 2010). Having an awareness of your emotional self can be useful in situations when emotions, yours or the patient's, begin to become heightened. Being self-aware and understanding the impact of your emotions on yourself and others can help when communication becomes challenging. Akerjordet and Severinsson (2004) argue that having the ability to empathise with patients is key to understanding their experience of suffering and distress. Van Dusseldorp et al. (2010, p556) state that *emotional intelligence is a prerequisite of key nursing skills like sensitivity, empathy, creativity, self awareness, self control and assertiveness.* Their research found that mental health nurses tended to have a higher than average level of emotional intelligence than the general population. This ability to be emotionally intelligent is described by Freshwater and Stickley (2004, p94) as the ability to *work in harmony with thoughts and feelings*.

If you are in a situation in which you begin to feel challenged, for example where you feel frightened, it is likely that if you are unaware of your emotions and your body language may portray how frightened you are. If your patient is also feeling frightened, the impact of this may be that the situation begins to escalate as your patient becomes more frightened rather than feeling safer. When emotions begin to dominate this stimulates the limbic system, the emotional part of the brain. In particular, stimulation of the amygdala may trigger a series of autonomic responses resulting in a 'fight or flight' response (Bear et al., 2007; Marieb and Hoehn, 2010). At these times the words may become less important than the non-verbal communication (Akerjordet and Severinsson, 2004).

Developing skills in emotional intelligence may help you form therapeutic relationships through self-awareness and the awareness of other emotions. Using effective clinical supervision and reflective practice can provide a safe environment in which to develop the skills required to recognise the impact of emotions on behaviours (Akerjordet and Severinsson, 2004; Freshwater and Stickley, 2004). Early recognition of your own emotions and potential responses in a situation will enable you to develop different strategies to provide compassionate care for your patients and their carers.

The National Collaborating Centre for Mental Health (2012) has identified that patients and carers want healthcare professionals to recognise the unique experiences of the individual. They also identified respect and trust as being key elements required to ensure a person-centred experience. Being aware of the impact of malignant social psychology and using this to further develop communication alongside emotional intelligence should help you develop a positive relationship with patients, carers and the interprofessional team.

Working with and caring for carers

It is important to recognise the part that carers may play in your patients' lives. Carers can suffer distress and may react to this in unexpected ways, perhaps by being angry or aggressive. This may not be how they usually behave: it may be a manifestation of their distress or previous negative experiences with services. We need to recognise and respect the important contribution that they make and consider how we can effectively communicate with them to support them and alleviate their distress.

At times this may be challenging, particularly if the patient doesn't want information shared. Even though a carer may be the chosen next of kin, this does not actually mean that she or he has any legal right to information. In the UK there is no legal definition of what this means, but patients who are subject to the Mental Health Act 1983 will have a 'nearest relative', which is defined using strict criteria (Barber et al., 2012; Mind, 2013; Murphy and Wales, 2013). It is important to be respectful both to your patients and their carers while maintaining confidentiality as outlined in *The Code* (NMC, 2008). You should not use 'confidentiality' as a way of avoiding having difficult conversations with carers. It is possible to talk to carers to help them understand what they can do to support the person they care for without breaching confidentiality (Mind, 2011).

Unpaid carers are estimated to save the NHS £119 billion a year (Brown, 2012) and yet there seems to be a lack of respect and compassion for this group, who are often more important to the patient than the healthcare professionals involved (Repper, 2012). Brown (2012, p2) outlines in the report for Carers UK that *instead of being supported, they often find their needs overlooked, they have to fight to get support and the support that is available is insufficient or of poor quality.* Brown also goes on the highlight that carers are not given either the information or the training to enable them to care for the patient well and safely.

Activity 5.7 — *Reflection*

- Go to the Patient Voices website at www.patientvoices.org.uk and listen to a couple of podcasts relating to the experiences of carers who are caring for someone with a mental health problem.
- Write down the thoughts and feelings you have while you are listening to these.
- Make a note of at least one thing you will do differently after listening to carers' experiences. Discuss this with you mentor and consider having it as one of your practice objectives.

As this activity is based on your own reflection, no outline answer is provided.

Your learning from this activity will depend on your chosen podcast. Listening to the real experiences of others will promote a compassionate response for the person telling the story. Compassion is a key component in demonstrating your values as a nurse. It forms one of the '6Cs' and is described as *how care is given through relationships based on empathy, respect and dignity* (Buckner and Yeandle, 2011, p13).

Activity 5.8 — *Critical thinking*

Mrs Smith's son, James, has been admitted to the acute unit where you are working. You hear a colleague say to her that they are unable to give her any information due to 'patient confidentiality', although currently James has no inclination to say either way if he wants his mother to have any information about his care. Mrs Smith is initially angry and then she becomes upset and leaves the clinical area.

Consider the following questions.

- Do you think that your colleague's actions were justified?
- Do you think Mrs Smith's reactions were understandable?
- Make a list of your justification for either agreeing or disagreeing with the actions and reactions.
- Is there anything that could have been done differently by your colleague?

An outline answer is provided at the end of the chapter.

Once you start thinking about confidentiality it becomes apparent that it is a complex issue, particularly when you have to take into consideration the often higher levels of risk for this patient group, their levels of vulnerability and the requirements of the Mental Health Act 1983 (amended 2007). More information about the complex nature of confidentiality in mental health nursing can be found in 'Outcomes of assessment' (Middlewick and Carpenter, 2013). You should also discuss these issues with your mentor as they are not straightforward. Using the experience of those around you will help you to develop confidence to support both your patients and their carers.

Chapter summary

Communication is usually at its most challenging when patients and their carers are in periods of distress. There may also be other physical health issues that contribute to this, some of which may be apparent and others hidden. Mental health nurses need the ability to piece the puzzle together so that they can work with patients, carers and the inter-professional team to ensure that there is a positive response. As a nurse you need to maintain a sense of curiosity about your patients so that, by exploring aspects of their lives, you will support them on their recovery journeys. All people have a story to tell if only we take the time to listen.

Activities: brief outline answers

Activity 5.1: Reflection (page 85)

You may have thought about challenges from your mental health clinical experiences from a diagnostic perspective, for example patients with a diagnosis of schizophrenia, depression, bipolar disorder, dementia or borderline personality disorder, or perhaps from a symptom perspective, for example being withdrawn, hearing voices, experiencing confusion, self-harming, feeling suicidal or being aggressive.

If you have been considering your patient more holistically you may also have thought about physiological issues such as hearing loss, visual difficulties, speech difficulties due to problems such as Parkinson's disease or cerebrovascular accident (CVA or stroke), or other factors such as being frightened or anxious.

You may have many other things on your list, but it is worth considering if you have tended to focus on mental health issues only or the symptoms you find challenging. You may also have highlighted some of the challenges of communicating with your patients' friends and carers.

Activity 5.5: Reflection (pages 90–1)

There could be any number of answers for this activity, and if you compared them to those of another person there may be some similarities, but it is highly likely that there would be a number of differences as we are all unique individuals.

Perhaps for keeping yourself well you said things such as eating well, sleeping, going out with friends, having enough money, having somewhere to live, feeling safe and secure, having a job you enjoy, having you hair cut, getting your legs waxed, going on holiday or keeping in touch with your family.

Some examples of things that might make you feel less good about yourself are people being rude, arguing with people close to you, worrying about money, being stressed, having too much to do and not enough time to complete the required tasks, not enjoying your job or not being in control of what is happening to you.

Activity 5.8: Critical thinking (page 94)

Do you think that your colleague's actions were justified?

It is of course true that nurses must maintain patient confidentiality; however, perhaps the delivery of this message could have been done in a more respectful and compassionate way. The nurse might also have explored how much James's mum knew about his current situation. Gaining the perspective of the carer can give you useful insights into how involved he or she is with the patient's care. It can also help you understand if the patient may be angry with the carer for perhaps instigating the involvement of services. Confidentiality is a complex area and is not as black and white as it at first appears. You need to ensure that you have a good understanding of your responsibilities as a student and then as a registered nurse.

Do you think Mrs Smith's reactions were understandable?

Yes, these reactions were completely understandable. Even if you are unable to give people information they still need to be treated with dignity and respect. It has been highlighted that carers can feel underprepared for their caring role and therefore we need to listen to their concerns and anxieties. This can also offer useful insights into what may be required to assist the patient on his or her recovery journey.

Is there anything that could have been done differently by your colleague?

Listening would have been a good start – trying to understand the situation from the patient's and carer's perspective. Your colleague should have enquired about how James was before he became unwell and gauged his mum's experiences of what has been helpful in the past.

Further reading

Kitwood, T (1997) *Dementia Reconsidered: The person comes first.* Buckingham: Open University Press.

This book gives an excellent insight into the meaning of person-centred care. Although the focus is on caring for people who have a diagnosis of dementia, the underlying principles are transferable to all areas of practice.

Murphy, R and Wales, P (2013) *Mental Health Law in Nursing.* London: Sage/Learning Matters.

This book is another practical guide to mental health law. It will help you unravel some of the complexities related to caring for people under the Mental Health Act.

Walker, S, Carpenter, D and Middlewick, Y (2013) *Assessment and Decision Making in Mental Health Nursing.* London: Sage/Learning Matters.

This book is a practical guide to the skills needed for assessing patients and making decisions resulting from assessments.

Useful websites

www.hearing-voices.org

The Hearing Voices Network offers recent experiences of people and will give you insight into the differing experiences that people have.

www.patientvoices.org.uk/index.htm

This website give you access to a wide range of personal experiences of patients, carers and professionals. It is particularly patients and carers who have been explored for this chapter. It gives you a real insight into what it is like to be on the receiving end of care and is well worth a visit.

Chapter 6
Cross-cultural communication
Julia Pelle

Chapter aims

By the end of this chapter you should be able to:

*   define cross-cultural communication;
*   identify barriers to cross-cultural communication in mental healthcare;
*   explore case study examples that infer the use of cross-cultural communication;
*   describe the effective communication strategies used in understanding culture and its potential impact on mental health.

Introduction

The previous chapter explored issues around cognitive impairment and the challenges of communication within mental healthcare. This chapter starts with a general introduction to cross-cultural communication in mental healthcare, followed by a review of the barriers to the delivery of cross-cultural communication. An overview of the effective communication strategies used in mental health practice will be discussed and the significant role of the mental health nurse in implementing these strategies will underpin the wider debate around cross-cultural communication. Any discussion about cross-cultural communication must also acknowledge one of the key drivers in its development, namely *transcultural nursing.*

In effective nursing practice we know that nurses need to deliver care remembering that at least some of their values, beliefs, attitudes, experiences and, indeed, cultural backgrounds will differ from those of the patients they care for (Spector, 2004).

Cross-cultural communication makes reference to three components of nursing practice. First is the subjective component, which focuses on nurses as cultural beings. This indicates that nurses need to develop self-awareness and insight into their own backgrounds. Lipson (1999) suggests that developing this level of one's own cultural awareness takes effort and time. Discovering differences in 'your' own worldview from that of others (peers, patients, carers) provides an opportunity to learn about human behaviour. Second, the objective component views the patient and communication characteristics that influence health, illness and care. The third component relates to the socioeconomic and political influences on healthcare. Lipson (1999) suggests that it is the immediate environment in a cross-cultural encounter that determines how nurses and clients interpret what is being communicated and what they express about themselves. For example, community mental health nursing may allow more detailed cultural assessment than accident and emergency care, psychiatric liaison or crisis intervention. There may also be regional differences in how cultural diversity is embraced.

The health policy document *Delivering Race Equality in Mental Health* (DH, 2005b) emphasised the need for mental health practice that addresses the health inequalities and institutional racism experienced by members of the black and minority ethnic communities, especially during their recovery from mental ill-health. Black and ethnic minority communities include people from Black African, African-Caribbean, South Asian and Chinese heritage, the Irish community, and Eastern European communities (to include Lithuanian, Latvian, Russian, Polish, Slovakian communities and the gypsy travelling community) (DH, 2005b). Bhui et al. (2013) state that *effective communication has proven more difficult to achieve where there are differences in culture and/or language of those delivering and receiving the health and social care.* Communication difficulties can be further exacerbated when both patient and professional meet and differences in age, gender, race/ethnicity, socioeconomic status or perceived power status exist. Lipson (1999) proposes that cross-cultural communication requires more than knowledge about various ethnic/cultural groups. It is a complex and interacting combination of knowledge, attitudes and skills.

This chapter examines one of the wider issues and the debate about the impact of culture on mental health and provides some critique of the issue of cross-cultural communication.

Gerrish et al. (1996) suggest that nursing professionals need to acquire and develop transcultural and communicative competence, which requires cultural competence – learning to understand the cultural values, behavioural patterns and rules for interaction in specific cultures. Bhui et al. (2013) suggest that nurses need to:

- identify and empathise with a patient from a different culture;
- understand symbolic and metaphorical language that varies by culture;
- understand differing expectations of healthcare professionals in different countries and cultures;
- appreciate the differences in illness perceptions and explanatory models of patients from different cultures.

Communication and culture are very closely linked; communication is a way to express culture, to begin to understand its meaning for the individual who lives in that culture, and to preserve the values, beliefs and practices that make up that culture.

Understanding how to communicate effectively with individuals from different cultural groups who are experiencing different mental health problems is an important part of mental health practice. As a mental health nurse you will need to use strong interpersonal skills that acknowledge a person's behaviour and responses as culturally driven and, while they may not match yours, culturally appropriate.

> ### Case study
>
> *Cynthia Obayomi is a 32-year-old Nigerian woman, admitted to the inpatient mental health unit via a referral from the Accident and Emergency department, with a history of bipolar disorder. Cynthia speaks a form of 'broken English' or what is more commonly known as 'pidgin English', not easily understood by staff caring for her. Cynthia relies on her aunt Gloria to translate for her but on this occasion she has become increasingly distressed that staff are talking with her aunt and not to her. Gloria informs staff that Cynthia has not taken any of her prescribed medication for the past week and has been observed spending long periods in her room, reciting parts of the Bible, writing copious Bible scriptures and refusing to eat anything, only occasionally leaving her room for a glass of water. Gloria was able to persuade Cynthia to come to hospital by telling her that they were going to the hospital chapel.*

Every patient is unique, but you will regularly be caring for people with some of Cynthia's problems. As you can see, her mental health issues are compounded by difficulties in communication.

The search for meaning: cross-cultural communication

Cross-cultural communication refers to how individuals from different cultural backgrounds communicate, in similar and different ways, and how they endeavour to communicate across cultures. Cross-cultural communication is increasingly important within the UK because of our multicultural population, the changing socioeconomic environment both nationally and internationally, the increase in globalisation and subsequent migratory patterns. Communities with different ethnicities may perceive mental health and well-being within the context of their cultural traditions.

Bhui et al. (2013) explain that cultural factors can affect therapeutic communication. This is important because they have the potential to compound inequalities in the social determinants of illness and to perpetuate inequalities in health and social care outcomes following contact with health and social care systems. Therapeutic communication can be central to reducing inequalities if done well.

Case study

Chandni is a 24-year-old woman who has been referred to the unit for a mental health assessment by her GP. She was accompanied by her husband to the unit and he informed the mental health nurse that his wife (who speaks very little English) stays in her room most of the day and ignores their two children. Sometimes when he gets home from work, he finds her in their bedroom crying, but she won't tell him what is wrong. Chandni, her husband and their two children recently migrated from Bangladesh and are currently living with her mother-in-law. At first, her husband believed her to be lazy, but now he is not sure. Throughout this meeting Chandni keeps her face covered and establishes no eye contact with the mental health nurse. However, she appears uncomfortable about being at this meeting and starts speaking in an angry tone of voice to her husband, who also starts to raise his voice.

Understanding cultural influences is important when you are conducting an initial mental health assessment. As we can see from the case study, culture influences how feelings are expressed and the type of verbal and non-verbal expressions that are appropriate.

Cross-cultural communication is said to comprise different aspects of interpersonal communication, which include verbal communication, non-verbal communication and intermeshing.

Activity 6.1   *Reflection*

Think back to a time when you were trying to communicate a piece of information to another person and he or she misinterpreted what you said. Note down any non-verbal modes of communication you used. Then, answer the following questions.

- How did it feel when the other person misinterpreted what you said?
- In what ways did you try to improve your communication so you could be better understood?

Discuss whether this helped the other person to understand you better.

As this activity is based on your own experience, no outline answer is provided.

Culture is inextricably linked to ethnicity, diversity and identity. It is essential that you know and understand the meaning of each of these terms and their link to cross-cultural communication. Please read through and familiarise yourself with the definition and descriptions below, before working on Activity 6.2.

Concept summary: Culture, ethnicity, race, diversity and identity

Culture comes from the Latin *cultura*, stemming from *colere*, meaning 'to cultivate'. Cultures can be understood as systems of symbols and meanings that lack fixed boundaries, that are constantly in flux and that interact and compete with one another (Spector, 2004).

Ethnicity is a cultural group's perception of themselves. It is a sense of belongingness and common social heritage demonstrated through an identity in common customs and traits.

Both culture and ethnicity may determine the way in which an individual or community chooses to access mental health and social care services, and how and when they choose to engage with service agencies. Cultural perceptions of mental illness and well-being can differ across and within different ethnic groups and subsequently influence self-perception and the degree of dependence on family and/or the mental health and social care services.

Race is now largely discredited as a classification of groups of people based on biological and physical similarities.

Diversity celebrates the differences between groups of people, according to their age, sex, culture, belief, disability, race, ethnicity, economic status, health status and so on. As such there is a diversity of health and social care settings that aim to meet the population diversity. Diversity is not 'equality'.

Identity is defined by Fernando (2010) as *a person's distinctive sense of uniqueness – of knowing who one is and is not.*

Campinha-Bacote (2002) developed a model of cultural competence to be used within the cultural context of health and social care services and the service user's perspective of well-being and illness. This model focuses on exploring the nurse's familiarity with the following five aspects.

- **Cultural desire** – the process of wanting to be culturally competent.
- **Cultural awareness** – a self-reflection of one's own biases.
- **Cultural knowledge** – obtaining information about different cultures.
- **Cultural skills** – conducting an assessment of cultural data of a patient.
- **Cultural encounters** – personal experiences of patients with different backgrounds.

Activity 6.2 — *Reflection*

Reflect on your own cultural background and answer each of the following questions.

- How would you describe your cultural heritage?
- What issues of culture, ethnicity and diversity are discussed in your everyday life in the UK?
- Name the different ethnic groups represented in the area where you live.

As this activity is based on your own knowledge, no outline answer is provided.

Identifying barriers to cross-cultural communication in mental healthcare

You will find that your patients and their families have varied perspectives, values, beliefs and behaviours regarding health and well-being. Health practitioners deal every day with diversity. This includes variations in recognition of signs and symptoms, thresholds of seeking professional care, ability to communicate symptoms to a provider who understands their meaning, ability to understand the agreed care management approach, expectations of care (including preferences of diagnostic and therapeutic procedures) and adherence to preventative measures and medications. These variations apply to patients with physical illness: imagine how this diversity is compounded by mental health issues.

Another reason for focusing on cross-cultural communication in mental health nursing is the mortality, morbidity and levels of risk in minority ethnic groups, those people with learning disabilities and older people. An extensive body of literature in the social sciences clearly indicates that achievement of an optimum level of health and the means to maintain well-being are culturally defined.

This section will now explore the more common barriers to cross-cultural communication that can occur in mental healthcare.

Common barriers to cross-cultural communication

We have seen that different ethnic groups may have different perceptions of mental illness and well-being from existing perceptions in the UK. Each cultural group perceives and subsequently defines health, illness and well-being in its own way. Many already prescribe the appropriate treatment in accordance to their own values and beliefs; an understanding of the patient's culture is therefore fundamental to health and social care. The professional also develops his or her own lens through which to view reality. This lens is refracted primarily through the professional's native culture, but this is then modified by professional socialisation, the culture of men or women, the culture of age and that of Western bio-medicine. These sets of beliefs and values intersect to form the clinician's blended worldview.

However, these can conflict with each other and with those of the patient and his or her family. Which template of patterns and behaviours is considered the 'right' way depends upon one's own worldview. Miscommunication is likely when the professional uses his or her Western bio-medical template of treating mental health problems as the right way, rather than one of several options or choices. The essences and rationalities of other cultural patterns are lost.

The culture-based system approach requires that practitioners are first aware of their own cultural beliefs and values in order to recognise when they may differ from those of the patient, and evaluate the patient's responses objectively. Both patient and professional bring their cultural views to the interaction.

Language and cultural differences

Language and cultural differences are potential barriers between patients, their families and mental health nurses (Cross and Bloomer, 2010). Where language barriers exist, using interpreters may not be enough, as word-for-word translation may not capture all the experience of mental illness (Cross and Bloomer, 2010). Interpreters need to have mental health training in order to be of the most benefit to both service users and mental health nurses. Another area of controversy is the fact that a number of patients may be bicultural – born to migrant parents from a country outside the UK, but having lived in the UK much of their lives. It is important not to assume that English is their first language.

Poor training and education in different cultural communities

It is a sad fact that the training of nurses is inadequate to enable them to employ cross-cultural communication in their everyday practice (Gerrish et al., 1996). When we fail to take socio-cultural factors into account this may lead to stereotyping, and in the worst cases biased or discriminatory treatment of patients based on race, culture, language proficiency or social status. A basic understanding of cultural diversity is the key to effective cross-cultural communications.

Case study

Mr Desmond Jamieson is a 72-year-old Caribbean man, with a diagnosis of late-onset Alzheimer's disease. His presenting symptoms include long- and short-term memory loss, feelings of agitation and anxiety, disrupted sleep patterns and an inability to make any rational decisions. Mr Jamieson lives with his wife Esther (his main carer) and their 34-year-old daughter Sandra, who has Down's syndrome, in a four-bedroom house. Mr Jamieson has become regularly incontinent of faeces and urine, and on two occasions in the last week he has turned the gas on and walked away from it, forgetting to turn it off. His wife Esther feels unable to leave him even when in the same house. The Jamiesons have another daughter, Janette, who does what she can to help in the care of her father, but she has a young family of her own and is not always able to help. The family are adamant that they do not want to place Mr Jamieson in a nursing home, stating that their cultural beliefs would never allow that to happen. Both Mr Jamieson and his wife are members of the local Baptist church and used to attend the African-Caribbean Association twice a week. Both have stopped going to church as Esther finds it hard to explain to friends what is happening and gets embarrassed by Mr Jamieson's behaviour.

| Activity 6.3 | *Critical thinking* |

- Look back to the earlier case study, about Cynthia (page 101). What cultural barriers exist between Cynthia and the staff, and between Cynthia and her aunt?
- Read again the case study about Desmond, above. How could the mental health nurse support this family with their carer roles and help them to maintain their beliefs about familial duty?
- Read the case study on Jing-Wei, below. What further information would a mental health nurse require to develop the assessment process with Jing-Wei? Describe some of the factors you would need to consider with a patient who is an adolescent. What aspects of Jing-Wei's cultural background would be helpful to further explore in your engagement with her?

An outline answer is provided at the end of the chapter.

Case study

Jing-Wei is a 15-year-old girl who has been admitted to the Child and Adolescent Mental Health Unit following a referral from the GP. Jing-Wei has been very low in mood, following receipt of her mock exam results in which she failed all subjects. She has two older brothers who are both at university and she lives at home with her parents who are visiting lecturers at the local university. The family migrated to the UK from China when Jing-Wei was 11 years old. During the family assessment, both parents expressed concern that Jing-Wei had lost a lot of weight over the past few weeks and does not speak to them any more; when she does speak, she is barely audible. Both parents, who are bilingual (Chinese/English), recall how it took some time for Jing-Wei to fit into secondary school life, but that they were very happy that she had picked up the English language so quickly.

Effective strategies for cross-cultural communication in mental health nursing

You will need a sound knowledge of how culture, ethnicity, race, diversity and identity influence mental well-being. This understanding is important for the development of the effective communication strategies that you will need while caring for patients from culturally diverse populations.

Maintaining cultural awareness as a mental health nurse

Before you can truly be engaged with using cross-cultural communication, it is necessary to address the 'culture of self'. This is where you examine your own sense of family tradition and upbringing and examine what mental illness, mental wellness and recovery mean to you within your own culture. It is important that you appraise the influence of values, beliefs and attitudes and recognise what your own culture, ethnicity, race and identity mean to you personally. This may mean attendance on tailored courses in cultural awareness that work towards cultural competence. Any such training should help engage mental health nurses with the diverse cultural groups/communities in their immediate area of health service delivery. You can then further develop your knowledge around the ethnic diversity of the health professional population, which can be an even more accessible form of learning in how to communicate in a cross-cultural way. However, without necessarily studying individual cultures and languages in detail, we must all learn how to better communicate with individuals and groups whose first language of choice does not match our own. The use of interpreters who also have an understanding of mental health problems and the mental health services provides a way forward.

Making effective use of interpreters

For some patients and health professionals the barrier to communication can be a lack of a common language and this is more likely to require the help of an interpreter. Having an interpreter for those clients whose language is different from yours fills an essential gap in communication, offers insight into the needs of the patient through the assessment process and gives information that increases access to mental health and social care services. The quality of the interpreter can impact on the quality of interaction between the patient and the mental health nurse. In many settings, no interpreter is available and you will have to rely on family members.

Involving family members

The importance of family carers' involvement in the overall care of their relatives with mental health problems is well recognised. However, several research studies have highlighted the subjective burden on carers of relatives with mental health problems. Some of this burden is made worse by poor information, advice and support by mental health services. An important part of your role as a mental health nurse is carrying out both patient and carer assessments; you will find out about carers' health needs, the coping strategies they currently use and how to improve their approach to caring. In order to establish a line of communication you will need to be very proactive in supporting carers by being approachable and available to answer any queries or concerns a family member may have. One of the areas where families feel neglected is in the provision of information on whom to contact out of hours and at weekends; another is feeling ill-prepared for the process of their relative being discharged back into their care. You need to maintain a reciprocal approach to communicating with carers through the caring process.

Establishing community-based networks

Drawing on knowledge of local voluntary or charity associations linked to different cultural and ethnic communities is another way of enhancing cultural awareness. Local council groups and community or town websites can be useful sources of information, especially if you are working in an area that is not the one in which you grew up.

Explore local ethnic community links, such as church leaders, local community associations and befriending groups. Consider establishing local community partnerships with different representatives, in order to support different patients who access the mental health services.

Negotiating staff training by local community representatives is another way to support cross-cultural communication. Do not neglect cultural knowledge among healthcare assistants, who may have insights based on their own ethnic backgrounds.

You can also use your influence by encouraging culturally sensitive work practices.

Case study

Ania Stanikowski is a 53-year-old Polish woman, with a diagnosis of schizoaffective disorder. This is her third episode in hospital for treatment. Ania was diagnosed two years after the sudden death of her husband Aleksy, from a heart attack. A past medical history indicates that Ania had three miscarriages and one stillbirth ten years ago, is currently unemployed and lives on her own in rented accommodation. She used to work as a healthcare support worker in a local nursing home. Ania and her husband migrated to the UK to earn enough money to return to a better quality of life in Poland. She is a devout Catholic, and recently during attendance at a service at her local Polish church was observed talking very loudly to herself, responding to voices that were telling her to 'go away, nobody wants you here, nobody loves you'. The priest contacted the emergency services, who located her community mental health nurse.

Religion can provide a way of coping with stressful life events and may help individuals reframe what is a larger-than-life problem into a more manageable situation. However, there are different forms of religious coping. For those individuals experiencing very high levels of emotional and mental distress, poor religious coping can increase their vulnerability and affect their physical and social well-being.

The mental health nurse needs to work with supporting Ania's current mental health needs and support her in looking at different treatment options. At a later date, because Ania is a devout Catholic, the mental health nurse can explore how her religion positively impacts her life – to understand its importance in Ania's everyday life.

The role of religion in mental health is complex, and you would do well to access some of the 'Further reading' materials listed at the end of this chapter to research this area more fully.

Developing culturally sensitive work practices

All mental health nurses must show compassion and empathy to both patients and their families. Where possible, you should arrange for a local community representative who knows the language and culture of the patient to 'meet and greet' the person when he or she arrives in the service. Provide reading materials in the language of the patient, and consider culturally appropriate food choices. Meeting the patient in this way will help to build the therapeutic alliance. Encourage family members and friends to visit the patient; when they are there, engage with them to learn more about the patient's cultural background.

Making effective use of clinical supervision

Because of the day-to-day challenges of being a mental health nurse in a constantly changing health and social care environment, it does take time to find out about every diverse and emerging culture. One of the ways you can address any problems with cross-cultural communication and share good practice ideas is through clinical supervision. Clinical supervision can help mental health nurses look at any cultural assumptions they may make in their interactions with patients in their care. Addressing these assumptions can help you to adjust your communication style to better assess patient needs (Bernard and Goodyear, 2004).

Ensuring ongoing training and education

Training in cultural awareness and cultural competency needs to form part of health and social care curricula and is a subject for lifelong learning. You need to be aware, though, that it is not enough to focus on your interpersonal communication skills, as the mere impact of mental illness can in itself have a devastating impact on a person's ability to communicate the aspects of their culture.

Chapter summary

This chapter has discussed the meaning of cross-cultural communication in general and how it relates to mental health nursing. The case study examples indicate some of the tacit links between culture, ethnicity, diversity and race that underpin the drive for effective cross-cultural communication. Definitions of culture, diversity and ethnicity vary and can be used interchangeably, but all agree on identifying with a social group with common ways of thinking, feeling and behaving. A personal awareness of your own culture, and the values you have as a result of your cultural identity, ethnicity and diversity, is a starting point for understanding transcultural health and social care issues. Stereotyping of families from different cultural/ethnic backgrounds can reduce contact with health and social care services and delay the process of recovery. The UK government has set guidance/policy for health and social care services to address inequalities in provision. It is important that mental health nurses communicating across cultures practise patience and work to increase knowledge and understanding of these cultures. This requires the ability to see that a person's own behaviours and reactions are often times culturally driven and, while they may not match our own, they are culturally appropriate. Generally speaking, patience, courtesy and a bit of curiosity go a long way. Equally important is the need to cultivate an environment of understanding and tolerance.

Activities: brief outline answers

Activity 6.3: Critical thinking (page 106)

Case 1: Cynthia

The cultural barriers between Cynthia and staff include:

- language differences;
- potentially different cultural background from that of the staff caring for her, indicated by religious practice and also having a country of birth outside the UK;
- potentially limited insight into her mental illness;
- actual tension and potential mistrust around staff talking to her aunt and not her.

The cultural barriers between Cynthia and her aunt include:

- Cynthia appears to be experiencing a relapse of her mental health problem;
- Cynthia's aunt may be older than her – potential generational differences;
- Cynthia may not trust her aunt as staff are communicating with her aunt and not her;
- Cynthia has been isolating herself at home – indicated by her staying in her room and not eating.

Case 2: Desmond

The mental health nurse needs to:

- assess how Esther feels about her carer role and explore how much support she has from her GP;
- identify if Esther has had a carer assessment of her needs;
- assess what caring Esther does for both her husband and her daughter Sandra; be aware that Sandra may also be helping her mother to care for Desmond;
- review what respite care Esther would like in order for her to carry out her carer role more effectively;
- propose and encourage a second appointment or meeting with Esther and her daughter Janette to consider how care could be more constructively shared;
- discuss what contact Esther has had with the Alzheimer's Society, which has information on local carer support groups she could attend.

Case 3: Jing-Wei

- In the first instance, as this is Jing-Wei's first time on an Adolescent Mental Health Unit, the role of the mental health nurse will be to reassure her and establish trust through discussing what has made her feel low in mood.
- Engaging with Jing-Wei may require the mental health nurse to start with questions about her hobbies, interests, etc. to establish a rapport.
- Other modes of engagement can be evoked through knowledge of Jing-Wei's cultural background. Learning a few words in Chinese with Jing-Wei's help could be a way to achieve this.
- Checking with Jing-Wei that she understands why she was referred to the adolescent unit, and what she knows about mental well-being, would also be a way to establish rapport.
- Later on in the development of trust the mental health nurse can ask Jing-Wei questions about why she thinks she failed all her exam subjects.
- Finding out from Jing-Wei if she felt low enough in mood not to want to live any more is an important conversation. The aim is to identify any risk she may pose to herself.

Further reading

Bhui, K, McCabe, R, Weich, S, Singh, S, Johnson, M and Szczpura, A (2013) THERACOM: A systematic review of the evidence base for interventions to improve therapeutic communications between black and minority ethnic populations and staff in specialist mental health services. *BioMedCentral: Systematic Reviews*, 2(1): Article No. 15.

Professor Kamaldeep Bhui is a Psychiatrist in Psychotherapy and contributes to the development of culturally capable mental health services in the UK. He has written a number of journal articles on culture, ethnicity and mental health.

Campinha-Bacote, J (2002) The process of cultural competence in the delivery of healthcare services: A model of care. *Journal of Transcultural Nursing*, 13(3): 181–4.

This article is written by Dr Josepha Campinha-Bacote, who developed a model of cultural competency in 1991 to be used within nursing practice. This provides a very useful overview of how the model can be applied to delivery of healthcare.

Cross, WM and Bloomer, MJ (2010) Extending boundaries: clinical communication with culturally and linguistically diverse mental health clients and carers. *International Journal of Mental Health Nursing*, 19(4): 268–77.

This is a very good article on cross-cultural communication in mental health with clients and carers that focuses on language differences.

Department of Health (DH) (2005) *Delivering Race Equality in Mental Health Care: An action plan for reform inside and outside services and the government's response to the independent inquiry into the death of David Bennett.* London: HMSO.

This is a Labour government policy on addressing the institutional racism highlighted in our UK mental health services and the action plan devised and in some areas implemented to address this.

Fernando, S (2010) *Mental Health, Race and Culture* (3rd edition). Basingstoke: Palgrave Macmillan.

This author has written and researched on a number of issues related to mental health, race and culture in the UK and this edition is a closer look at cultural beliefs, values and perceptions of mental health and well-being, as well as the political issues that encompass healthcare.

Gerrish, K, Husband, C and Mackenzie, J (1996) *Nursing for a Multi-ethnic Society.* Buckingham: Open University Press.

This book gives a very helpful nursing perspective on multicultural aspects of delivering professional nursing care, and gives some background to the ethnicity of health professionals and the cultural and ethnic considerations of different black and minority ethnic communities.

Lipson, JG (1999) Cross-cultural nursing: the cultural perspective. *Journal of Transcultural Nursing*, 10(1): 6.

Professor Emeritus Julienne Lipson has written widely on cross-cultural communication in nursing and this commentary gives an overview of the nurse as a 'cultural being'.

Spector, RE (2004) *Cultural Diversity in Health and Illness* (6th edition). Englewood Cliffs, NJ: Pearson-Prentice Hall.

This is a very useful textbook on culture, ethnicity and diversity – it focuses on a USA population but includes key cultural traditions of different ethnic communities.

Useful websites

www.afiya-trust.org

This is a national charity that aims to reduce inequalities in health and social care for people from different ethnic groups in the UK. This is a very good resource for reviewing the experiences of carers from black and ethnic minority (BME) communities; the site has a number of publications related to BME carers.

www.dh.gov.uk

This is the Department of Health website where policy information on carers can be accessed by typing in the search term 'carers'. Both past and current government carer policies are included.

www.justice.gov.uk/human-rights

This is the Ministry of Justice website where you can access human rights policy and associated documents.

www.kingsfund.org.uk

This is a charity with a primary aim of looking at how government policy and the health and social care services can improve patient care in the UK. It organises conferences and events that help wider participation in discussing these issues. One of its many topic areas includes mental health; it has conducted a number of research studies and is a good resource for health and social care publications.

www.rcn.org.uk/development/learning/transcultural_health/communication

This is a direct link to a module devised by the RCN to enhance interpersonal communication skills by giving you knowledge of the different ethnic groups in Great Britain and developing your cultural awareness, sensitivity and competence in supporting the health and social care needs of vulnerable individuals.

Chapter 7
Communication with carers as partners in care

Julia Pelle

NMC Standards for Pre-registration Nursing Education

This chapter will address the following competencies:

Domain 2: Communication and interpersonal skills

6. All nurses must take every opportunity to encourage health-promoting behaviour through education, role modelling and effective communication.

6.1 **Mental health nurses** must foster helpful and enabling relationships with families, carers and other people important to the person experiencing mental health problems. They must use communication skills that enable psychosocial education, problem-solving and other interventions to help people cope and to safeguard those who are vulnerable.

NMC Essential Skills Clusters

This chapter will address the following ESCs:

Cluster: Care, compassion and communication

1. As partners in the care process, people can trust a newly registered graduate nurse to provide collaborative care based on the highest standards, knowledge and competence.

By the first progression point:

1. Articulates the underpinning values of *The Code: Standards of conduct, performance and ethics for nurses and midwives* (NMC, 2008).

By the second progression point:

6. Forms appropriate and constructive professional relationships with families and other carers.

By entry to the register:

12. Recognises and acts to overcome barriers in developing effective relationships with service users and carers.

13. Initiates, maintains and closes professional relationships with service users and carers.

continued . . . •••

Cluster: Organisational aspects of care

9. People can trust the newly registered graduate nurse to treat them as partners and work with them to make a holistic and systematic assessment of their needs; to develop a personalised plan that is based on mutual understanding and respect for their individual situation promoting health and well-being, minimising risk of harm and promoting their safety at all times.

By the second progression point:

5. Contributes to care based on an understanding of how the different stages of an illness or disability can impact on people and carers.

10. People can trust the newly registered graduate nurse to deliver nursing interventions and evaluate their effectiveness against the agreed assessment and care plan.

By the second progression point:

1. Acts collaboratively with people and their carers enabling and empowering them to take a shared and active role in the delivery and evaluation of nursing interventions.

By entry to the register:

6. Provides safe and effective care in partnership with people and their carers within the context of people's ages, conditions and developmental stages.
9. Evaluates the effect of interventions, taking account of people's and carers' interpretation of physical, emotional and behavioural changes.

Chapter aims

By the end of this chapter you should be able to:

* define the terms 'partnership' and 'carer';
* list the different types of carer in mental health;
* identify the needs of those who care for individuals with mental health problems;
* discuss the role of the mental health nurse in partnership with carers;
* describe the advantages and disadvantages of a partnership between mental health practitioners and carers for clients/service users.

Introduction

The best and most beautiful things in the world cannot be seen or even touched – they must be felt with the heart.

(Helen Keller, 1880–1968)

Reviewing the meaning of 'carer' and how carers work in partnership with mental health nurses is the theme of this chapter. In Chapter 6 we discussed cross-cultural communication and its importance in how healthcare is delivered effectively, especially in mental healthcare. In this chapter we explore how carers, usually family members or friends, become important in supporting the delivery of health and social care to different client groups. Most family members or friends do not see themselves as carers, but rather see their role as part of family responsibility, and their commitment to take care of a spouse or partner 'in sickness and in health'.

We will define 'partnership' in the context of mental health and social care practice. As a nurse, you will take a 'partnership approach' to involving carers in care for others; this means you will assess the health and social care needs of carers, who may have the burden of caring over long periods of time, as well as trying to adjust to their role as carer. You need to be aware of the difficulties some groups in society have in accessing support from health and social care services; because of this you will need to focus on carer groups that may not be reached due to stigma, social exclusion and discrimination. Such groups include young carers, carers who are economically disadvantaged, carers from black and ethnic minority communities and carers from lesbian, gay, bisexual and transgendered communities.

Case study

Anna is a 28-year-old woman, who cares for her older sister Beth (32 years old), who was diagnosed with bipolar disorder ten years ago. Anna took on the full-time care of Beth six years ago, following the death of both their parents in a serious car accident. Recently Beth has refused to take her medication and has become increasingly sexually disinhibited and verbally aggressive towards Anna. Anna and Beth share the same home and Anna has been unable to get a good night's sleep, finding herself worrying about her sister and how to encourage her to take her medication; she does not want her sister to go back into hospital, as Beth has had several bad experiences as an inpatient, which leaves Anna feeling guilty and angry at the same time. Anna, who by this time is feeling very distressed and desperate to gain some control of the situation, contacts Beth's community mental health nurse and asks for help with getting a break from her caring role.

This case study describes the impact on a carer's health when caring for a person with mental health problems. This chapter will discuss the impact of caring on those who care for people with mental health problems. Research on carers tends to focus on two areas of burden, namely objective burden (the effect of caring on the household, which includes taking care of daily tasks for the cared-for person) and subjective burden (the extent to which the carer perceives the burden of care). Later in this chapter we will look at how, as a mental health nurse, you can communicate with the diverse group of carers to enhance the partnership relationship.

What is a carer?

First, let us be clear about what we mean by a carer.

The Carers Trust (2012) defined a carer as:

> *someone of any age, who provides unpaid support to family and friends who could not manage without this help. This could be caring for a relative, partner or friend who is ill, frail, disabled or who has mental health or substance misuse problems. Anyone can become a carer. Carers come from all walks of life and all cultures.*

The first stage in your partnership with carers is to establish who is the primary carer of a service user/patient. The primary carer is usually the person who spends the most time with an individual. Primary carers may be able to tell you just how the patient's mental health problem manifests in the home environment and in the community, which is information vital to your assessment. Your early contact with the primary carer is also an opportunity to review what support the primary carer is likely to need in order to continue with his or her caring role. For example, he or she may need more education about the signs and symptoms of mental health problems and information on support organisations. Be sure that you also acknowledge all other family members and friends who play a secondary carer role.

What is partnership?

In order to understand how carers can work in partnership with health and social care services we also need a meaningful definition of what 'partnership' actually entails. Hatfield (1994) gives a meaningful definition of partnership through relating this to collaboration:

> *Collaboration means shared problem definition, shared decision-making, and shared responsibility with final decisions reflecting a balance of the needs of all those involved. It means working with people rather than doing things to them.*

The partnership relationship between carers and health and social care professionals brings benefits but also has its challenges, and these are noted in Table 7.1.

Activity 7.1   *Critical thinking*

Look at the points listed under the 'Challenges' column in Table 7.1. Think about how you as a mental health nurse could address these in clinical practice. If possible, discuss these issues with a colleague or in groups of two to four.

An outline answer is provided at the end of the chapter.

Benefits	Challenges
Can result in improved patient care outcomes.	Feeling like a go-between for the cared-for person and professionals.
Can give valuable insight into how the patient responds to treatment at home.	Inconsistent service provision between different health and social care agencies.
Can give a more detailed assessment of the impact of mental health problems.	
Relationships can be further enhanced between carer and patient.	Lack of skills in identifying mental health problems; needs training in how to help patient manage triggers of illness and in knowing when to intervene effectively.
Advance directives can improve communication and partnership between carers and staff, because they ensure agreement about each person's role in caring for a patient.	Health and social care professionals do not always recognise the psychological and physical needs of carers.
	Too much focus on medication and limited discussion on other non-medication interventions, e.g. counselling and psychotherapy.
	Not all carers want to be in a carer role.
	Misconception of 'confidentiality and privacy policies' by both professionals and carers.
	Professionals do not have time to involve carers.
	Carers experience as much stigmatisation as patients.
	Increased subjective burden of care.
	Change of diagnosis.
	Differential explanations for why mental illness occurs, i.e. biological, environmental, psychological etc.
	Perception of family carer as actual or potential cause of mental health problems.
	Cultural differences in perception of family caring between carers and professionals.

Table 7.1: Benefits and challenges in partnership

Identifying the needs of carers

Considering the needs of carers is a fundamental part of working collaboratively with them. The following section will outline some of the main areas that you need to be mindful of when developing a working relationship with carers.

A need for information about mental health problems

For many carers there are several issues around the types of information they need to fulfil their caring role. In the first instance, carers of individuals with mental health problems require information that tells them about the signs and symptoms of mental illness. The unexpected changes in persona and unpredictability of mood and behaviour they experience in the persons they care for can leave carers feeling shocked, anxious and angry; this can lead to a breakdown in the social relationship and ultimately delay the adaptation to their role as carers.

You will also need to be able to explain carefully any terms of the Mental Health Act 1983, and its amendments, that may apply to your patients. Carers can become confused, dismayed and intimidated by their observation of the use of this Act, particularly in the care of their relatives or friends, and they should feel able to receive advice from you on these issues.

Expectations of mental health and social care services

Often carers have expectations about mental health and social services that are unrealistic: as we know, the reality of the health and social care environment is increasingly governed by a range of national policies. For example, carers may feel they have to wait too long before there is any action on the statutory care of their relatives or friends. It may be your role to explain how the system works, and give them realistic expectations. You can also help by giving information on local carer support groups or respite care intervention (DH, 2012).

Issues of confidentiality

Carers can become concerned by the lack of information they struggle to receive from health professionals in relation to the care of their relatives or friends, which leads to more frustration and can also increase the burden of caring.

Scenario

Imagine you are nursing Pranav, who has paranoid schizophrenia, and usually lives with his father, Shrey, a widower. Pranav has been in an acute inpatient mental health ward for the last two weeks since experiencing a relapse in his mental state. Shrey rings the ward to ask if Pranav has been taking his medication and could nursing staff check. (Pranav has been phoning Shrey at home several times in the day and then hanging up the phone.) The nurse who speaks to Shrey on the phone says she is unable to relay this information because of the rules on confidentiality. She also says that Pranav does not want any information to be shared with his father. Shrey gets very angry, as he is aware that Pranav can conceal his medication when no one is looking, and staff may not be aware of this.

As a mental health professional you are guided by specific trust policies on confidentiality, which can be a barrier to partnership working with carers. We know that carers would like to have a more partnership approach to the sharing of information; they would like to know about matters discussed in Care Programme Approach (CPA) meetings, the ongoing assessment of patients, their plans of care and information about medication management.

Access to the full range of mental health service provision

Research has highlighted several issues you need to understand. Carers have expressed their worries about whether their relatives are receiving full access to all the mental health and social services. Furthermore, carers have experienced not being attended to by mental health and social services. They lacked care and information in the difficult life situation. When their relatives were discharged, the responsibility was again transferred to them, often without any follow-up by the mental health and social care services. Carers complained of feeling more like silent partners in their interaction with mental health and social care services and they also felt undervalued by local services.

Taking care of their own needs: carer assessments

We have already seen that the assessment of carers is an important starting point for you in working with family carers. Carer assessments help people identify the effects of caring on their everyday lives, helping them focus on their own needs. Such assessments are usually carried out by the local social services department. The carer assessment can help local social services to determine what support they can offer carers. However, as there are different perceptions of carers and their responsibilities, there is also a variety of ideas around how services should interact with carers, and ultimately how a carer assessment is conducted. For instance, some services favour interventions that support carers to continue their caring role for as long as possible, whereas others consider service support should consist of any action that helps carers to take up or decide not to take up, to continue or to end their carer role.

Activity 7.2	*Decision making*

How would you carry out an assessment of the health and social care needs of carers in mental healthcare? Support your answer with evidence from the wider literature; please refer to the 'Further reading' section of this chapter.

An outline answer is provided at the end of the chapter.

Different types of carer

Within a family of carers there can be further diversity of caring role where care is shared between various family members. There may be parental carers, spousal carers, sibling carers, or young and older carers. Remember also that carers may also be experiencing their own health problems related to old age, and some may have mental health problems of their own. It is common for carers to have financial worries because they have had to give up paid employment, which can increase the burden of caring. Certainly, a group of carers who can go unnoticed within mental health and social services include young carers, older carers, carers from black and minority ethnic communities, and carers who are lesbian, gay, bisexual or transgendered.

Young carers

Although there has been legislation recognising young carers and guidance for different health and social care agencies on how to support them, many go unnoticed within the health, social and education services. Only small numbers of young carers are being identified and assessed. This has been further compounded by the blurring of boundaries of responsibility between adult and child services (Social Care Institute for Excellence (SCIE), 2005). Young carers experience psychological, social and physical health problems, which may manifest themselves during their time in school. Many young carers have highlighted the importance of and welcomed the Young Carer Projects that have been introduced to support them, but these are not consistently provided in every geographical location of the UK.

Case study

Adam is 16 years old and has been caring for his mother (Sarah), who has been diagnosed with clinical depression for the last ten years. Sarah has to take prescribed antidepressants every day to manage her depression and just recently has begun to attend the community treatment team for one-hour sessions in cognitive behaviour therapy (CBT). Adam has the responsibility of ensuring that his mother takes her medication and goes to her psychiatrist/community mental health nurse appointments and her CBT sessions. Adam is in his final year of his GCSEs and has found it increasingly difficult to check that his mother takes her medication. Sarah has already refused to attend her CBT sessions on two occasions. Adam has noticed a change in his mother's behaviour and she has started to say things like, 'You would be better off without me ...'.

Adam has found it hard to cope with his mother's depression and has taken some time off school in order to keep her safe.

Older carers

Older carers may have their own physical health problems related to ageing to deal with, in addition to the burden of caring for a relative or friend, which has its own psychological, social and physical concerns. Some carers who are older and in poor health worry about what will happen to their loved ones when they are no longer around to care for them.

Case study

Ruth is 68 and has responsibility for caring for her husband, Donald, 75, who has a diagnosis of Alzheimer's disease. Ruth has recently been diagnosed with breast cancer and is worried about what might happen to her husband, who requires full care for all of his physical and cognitive health needs, as her own illness takes its course. They have two children who live quite far away, and who visit on special occasions only. Ruth, who is being attended to by the cancer care services, has been advised by the nurses to seek more support from her GP and her family.

Activity 7.3	*Team working*

Read through the two previous case studies.

- In the case of Adam, who are the agencies and services that need to get involved in the support of Adam in his carer role?
- In Ruth's case, what help does Ruth need from the mental health nurse in planning for the future care of both herself and her husband Donald?

An outline answer is provided at the end of the chapter.

Black and minority ethnic carers

While carers from BME communities have very similar experiences to those of other carers, each ethnic group of the BME community has its own unique experiences of caring, some of which are reflected in the journeys they go through with the family members they care for (NBCCWN, 2008). BME carers also experience additional barriers, including gaining equal access to mental health and social care; cultural, language, ethnic group and dialectical differences; the psychological and socio-economic impact of their migration history to the UK; perceptions of care, caring and mental health; increased poor health; and institutional racism. Despite recognition of the importance of family carers in the recovery of their sick relatives, this role has been largely ignored in BME communities.

Scenario

Imagine you are the mental health nurse caring for Marlon, who has been detained under the Mental Health Act 1983. His sister Monique is a 28-year-old 'new' carer for her older brother, who has a diagnosis of schizophrenia. Monique has only recently migrated to the UK from Martinique in the Caribbean and was unaware of the severity of her brother's illness until she experienced a rapid change in his behaviour at home while they were eating dinner. Monique had to telephone the police and subsequently her brother was detained under the Mental Health Act 1983 and transferred to the local inpatient unit where you work. The whole experience has left Monique feeling guilty, frightened for the future and worried that she will not be able to work in her job as a legal secretary and manage the care of her brother as well.

What reassurance can you give to Monique about her role as a carer so far? First, you will need to acknowledge the role Monique has as a carer. As Monique's brother has an enduring mental health problem, he will be cared for under the provision of the Care Programme Approach. He will be allocated to a Care Coordinator who can support Monique to care for her brother in several ways. She will have the opportunity to express how she feels about the experience of caring, and will be given relevant information about her brother's mental health problem and the process of treatment outlined for him during his stay in hospital. You can help in assessing whether Monique is happy to continue her carer role, and review with Monique where she needs support in caring for her brother when he comes out of hospital. Make sure Monique knows about her rights as a carer who is in employment, and discuss her rights as a carer to financial and respite support.

Lesbian, gay, bisexual and transgendered carers

A number of LGBT carers have had experience of discrimination and stigmatisation in their lifetimes. This may be because of the higher incidence of mental health problems in this community compared to their heterosexual counterparts; as such they may experience stigmatisation in relation to both their sexual orientation and their mental health (DH, 2008b).

> ### Case study
>
> *Darren, who is a 45-year-old gay man, has been a carer for his partner Jamie for the last three years. Jamie is 31 years old, and was diagnosed with bipolar disorder when he was 28 years old following a coming out period where he told his family about his sexuality. Darren has noticed that Jamie, who is taking medication for his bipolar disorder, has recently been increasingly aggressive towards him, both verbally and physically. Darren suspects Jamie is taking illicit drugs, which might explain his recent behaviour, but does not know who to turn to for help.*

Darren needs to contact Jamie's care coordinator (who can be any allocated member of the multidisciplinary team, for example a consultant psychiatrist and or community mental health nurse (CMHN)) and explain exactly what has happened and his own fears about his own safety. Jamie should be registered with a GP (who could also be the main care coordinator), and Darren should contact Jamie's GP and provide as much information as possible about Jamie's present mental and physical health status. Another person Darren could contact is the nurse/psychiatrist on call in the local acute inpatient mental health hospital in order to get further advice and support. It is a requirement of mental health and social care services to support and assess a person who is experiencing a mental health crisis. In addition, Darren can contact the crisis resolution and home treatment (CRHT) team (based in community mental health services) to help and support him with his brother. These teams are usually community based and details of their contact numbers should have already been given to Darren as Jamie's carer. Some mental health service provision may be accessible through the accident and emergency (A&E) department – where there may be a liaison psychiatric service – however, they will only assess individuals who are being treated by A&E staff, or have already been admitted to a general hospital for a physical health problem. Darren should also be prepared for the possibility of the local police services becoming involved, particularly where Jamie may pose a risk to himself or others.

Activity 7.4   *Reflection*

- Describe how you might feel when someone you know, either a close friend or family member, is admitted to a hospital for treatment.
- Focusing on this experience, discuss and write down the different ways in which one person can give care to another.
- Describe the benefits for friends and family who care for others.
- How might a carer feel when his or her family member or close friend has been admitted to a psychiatric hospital for treatment?

An outline answer is provided at the end of the chapter.

Acknowledging different types of carer

It is important that nurses acknowledge the different types of carer in mental healthcare. This is because different types of carer have their own support needs; for example, parental carers may need more support adjusting to the fact that their usual parental role for their children will be extended to include a more proactive role, where an adult offspring may remain very dependent on them from childhood into later adulthood. Spousal carers may need support with how best to maintain intimacy in their relationships with loved ones who have mental health problems. Young carers may find their social lives change as they have to care for parents, who are dependent on them to care for younger children in the family, take on responsibility for most household chores and ensure their parents attend hospital/GP appointments.

Information that carers need

As a nurse you are well placed to help carers access the information they need. This is a checklist of the kinds of information most beneficial to carers in their carer role.

- Information on how to recognise signs and symptoms of mental illness.
- Information on whom to contact in the health and social care services when they are unable to cope with changes in cared-for persons' mental states.
- Information on where they can seek support for themselves.
- Information on their rights to care for themselves and right to support in their carer role.
- Information on any financial aid they can access and or how to manage finances when caring.
- Learning what approaches they can use to intervene effectively when their relatives or cared-for persons are unwell.

Activity 7.5   *Critical thinking*

- Why is it important for carers to know what their rights are in the caring process?

An outline answer is provided at the end of the chapter.

Chapter summary

Consider all the key focus areas of this chapter by reading through the case study examples given and reflecting on this for your practice placement experiences. What becomes immediately evident is that carers have quite specific needs, some of which are generic to all and others that are very individual. There are several opportunities during the process of assessment of a patient for the carer to be jointly assessed and also involved in the process of care. Mental health nurses can assess how much carers do in terms of caring for their relatives or friends, and work with carers as allies in the construction of detailed assessments of patients' needs. A process of joint decision making around care planning and communication of the range of interventions that both patients and carers can access from the beginning of making contact with mental health services can prove effective in ensuring a better recovery for patients and carers feeling well supported and valued.

Activities: brief outline answers

Activity 7.1: Critical thinking (page 116)

There is no absolute right answer to all of these challenges and much will depend on the local mental health service policies and government guidance as well as the individual patient and carer.

Challenge	**Potential ways to address this challenge in clinical practice**
Feeling like a go-between for the cared for person and professionals.	Where the cared-for person has given consent, organise an open meeting between carer, cared-for person and professionals.
Inconsistent service provision between different health and social care agencies.	Help the carer and cared-for person establish who in the mental health and social care services can be the main care coordinator of their care, e.g. a GP, social worker, mental health nurse or psychiatrist, and this person can be the liaison between different health and social care services.
Lack of skills in identifying mental health problems; needs training in how to help patient manage triggers of illness and in knowing when to intervene effectively.	Psycho-education by peer trainers, mental health and social care professionals, and mental health organisations, e.g. MIND, RETHINK etc.

Health and social care professionals do not always recognise the psychological and physical needs of carers.

It is important here to signpost carers to how they can have their own health and social care needs assessed – this could take place via the social services department or their GPs.

Too much focus on medication and limited discussion on other non-medication interventions, e.g. counselling and psychotherapy.

Open discussion with cared-for person and all health and social care professionals involved in his or her care.

Not all carers want to be in a carer role.

Misconception of 'confidentiality and privacy policies' by both professionals and carers.

The mental health services and social care services need, as soon as possible, to discuss the implications of the confidentiality of information policies within the Trust.

Professionals do not have time to involve carers.

Staff training on carer roles and carer training on the set-up of mental health and social services.

Carers experience as much stigmatisation as patients.

Information on carer support groups to help individual carers feel less stigmatised. Education on mental health problems.

Increased subjective burden of care.

Encourage a more open discussion with GP. Discuss the possibility of carer assessment.

Change of diagnosis.

Education on mental health problems and why diagnoses may change over time.

Differential explanations for why mental illness occurs, i.e. biological, environmental, psychological etc.

Education on the different mental health problems and what are considered (a) common mental health problems and (b) enduring mental health problems.

Perception of family carer as actual or potential cause of mental health problems.

Cultural differences in perception of family caring between carers and professionals.

Staff training on cultural issues in mental health practice.

Activity 7.2: Decision making (page 119)

An important point to make is that most carers have a legal right to have an assessment of their own health and social care needs. For carers of persons with mental health problems, they have a right to an assessment of their own needs if the people they care for have health and social care provision under the Care Programme Approach (CPA). The CPA is a particular approach to assessing, planning and reviewing a person's mental health and social care needs. A CPA is usually provided for persons with severe mental health problems.

- It is important to ascertain how long the friend or family member has been caring for his or her relative.
- Establish if the person is happy in the role of carer. Many family members believe that it is their duty to care for their relative without being fully aware of the task they are undertaking.
- If the carer is happy to continue – is there anything he or she would like to change to make the caring role easier?
- Do others also share the caring role with this carer? If yes, find out who the other people are.
- Find out if the carer has any physical or mental health problems of her or his own.
- Does the caring role impact on other social relationships?
- Is the carer currently in full- or part-time work and how does he or she fulfil the caring role as a result?

- Does the carer want more time to him- or herself? This indicates possible times when he or she may need respite.
- Would the carer be interested in doing training around mental health, legal aspects of mental health, recognising signs and symptoms of illness, information on medication used in mental illness etc.?
- Find out if the carer is aware of the different carer support services he or she can access in the caring role. This could include financial support, social care support and having an annual health check with a GP.
- Indicate resources from the literature, e.g. UK carer policies.

Activity 7.3: Team working (page 121)

Case study: Adam

Young people under the age of 18 are entitled to a carer assessment of their needs. This is usually carried out by the local Children's Department under the provisions of the Children Act 1989. Under the Carers and Disabled Children Act 2000, carers of 16 and 17 years of age can have a carer assessment.

- School nurse – a school nurse can review the impact of caring on Adam's everyday life, including school work, and also signpost Adam to a social worker in the local Children's Department of the local council for a carer assessment. An important part of this process involves communication with the parents and other family members – there are local school policies for young carers that stipulate a protocol for acknowledging young carers and how to support them.
- Youth workers and young person project workers may also be part of the local council provision and can signpost a young person to a social worker in the Children's Department.

Case study: Ruth

- Ruth needs to be encouraged to make an appointment to meet with her GP and discuss the support she needs. As Ruth has had contact with different services it may be that her GP is already aware of her carer role and her personal health needs. However, the GP can refer Ruth to Social Services for a carer assessment.
- As part of the carer assessment the GP can provide a subsequent report on her physical and emotional health and social care needs and the carer role she has for her husband.
- Also the GP should have access to the different local carer groups/organisations and information about the Macmillan Nurses.
- Ensuring that Ruth has regular health checks, and addressing any financial or respite support she needs, are also areas the GP can assist her with.

Activity 7.4: Reflection (page 123)

How you might feel if a close friend or family member is admitted to hospital:

- anxious;
- worried;
- fearful about going into a hospital to either accompany or see your friend/relative.

The different ways a person can give care to another include:

- being there and listening to the person's concerns about his or her health;
- recognising when the person is unwell;
- encouraging the person to seek further advice about how unwell he or she is feeling;
- helping the person gather information about her or his illness;
- accompanying the person to a GP or other health professional as a way of supporting her or him.

The benefits for friends and family who care for others include:

- a sense of achievement and fulfilment;
- developing a closer relationship with the cared-for person;
- more self-awareness of their own personal strengths in challenging situations around caring.

How carers might feel when their family members or close friends have been admitted to a psychiatric hospital for treatment could include the following.

- Carers may feel a sense of personal failure for not being able to cope with their relatives/friends at home and now those persons have been admitted to hospital.
- Some carers may, in fact, feel a strong sense of relief that someone else is able to take over the care of their relatives as they may have been struggling.
- Carers may experience a fear of leaving their relatives in what can be a very strange and initially quite threatening hospital environment. This fear can also be related to their observation of other patients in the ward environment. Other patients may be experiencing more severe aspects to their mental health problems, which may make them appear frightening. There may also be fears about treatment approaches in this environment, particularly where the administration of antipsychotic medication is concerned.
- Carers may experience an overwhelming sense of guilt.
- Carers may in their early caring role experience a sense of hopelessness and despair. This becomes more apparent when they are unable to perceive recovery for their relatives.
- Anger may be justifiably directed at mental health and social care services where there are perceived and actual lapses in the care of their relatives.

Activity 7.5: Critical thinking (page 124)

It is important for carers to know what their rights are in the caring process because:

- there is more chance of getting needs assessed and receiving more tailored individual support in the caring role;
- if there are young carers in the family, this is likely to mean that their well-being is addressed and there is an opportunity to offer support that meets their needs;
- it may inform carers about other policy and Acts that can further support them in their carer role, e.g. the Employment Act 2002 and the Carers (Equal Opportunities) Act 2004;
- it may also mean that carers are eligible for receiving direct payments issued by local authorities for carers and the cared-for person can purchase specific health and social care;
- it gives carers rights to NHS care under the NHS Constitution written in January 2009 and updated in March 2012.

Further reading

Department of Health (DH) (2004) *Carers Equal Opportunities Act.* London: HMSO.

This Act sought to ensure that carers were identified and informed of their rights, that their need for education, training, employment and leisure were taken into account, and that public bodies gave the necessary support to carers.

Department of Health (DH) (2008) *Carers at the Heart of the 21st Century: Families and communities.* London: HMSO.

This was a Labour government carer strategy, which was to update the 1999 carer policy and develop a national information helpline for carers; introduce a new training programme for carers; and invest further funding in councils to provide emergency care cover.

Department of Health (DH) (2010) *Recognised, Valued and Supported: Next steps for the Carers Strategy*. London: HMSO.

This was a Coalition government policy dealing with four priority areas: early identification of carers; increasing opportunities for carers to fulfil their educational and employment potential; personalising support of carers; and helping carers to manage their mental and physical health needs.

Department of Health (DH) (2012) *Caring for Our Future: Reforming care and support*. London: HMSO.

This was a Coalition government White Paper, outlining changes to how care and support will be delivered to individuals. In this paper it is indicated that carers will be given more support, with particular reference to their health needs.

Hatfield, A (1994) The family's role in caregiving and service delivery, in Lefley, H and Wasom, M (eds) *Helping Families Cope with Mental Illness*. Newark, NJ: Harwood Academic Publishers.

This useful textbook highlights the previous research into the impact of mental illness on family carers, reviewing medication and non-drug therapy interventions, and different populations of service users with enduring mental health problems.

National Black Carers and Carers Workers Network (NBCCWN) (2008) *Beyond We Care Too: Putting black carers in the picture*. London: Afiya Trust.

This is a detailed report presenting survey results of the experience of carers from the black and minority ethnic (BME) communities living in the UK. It reviews a number of areas of concern for carers and makes recommendations for how health and social care can be developed to help and support carers from these communities.

Social Care Institute for Excellence (SCIE) (2005) *SCIE Research Briefing 11: The health and well-being of young carers*. London, SCIE.

This is a report summarising the evidence from the research literature on the health and well-being of young carers in the UK.

Useful websites

www.ageuk.org

This is a joint collaboration between Age Concern and Help the Aged to support patients and their carers in later life. This website has a professional homepage section, which gives more discussion around key issues in older persons' health, e.g. dementia, and also gives further information about the latest government publications for later-life care.

www.carers.org

This is the Carers Trust, which includes The Princess Royal Trust for Carers and Crossroads Care. This website offers support, information and advice for carers, through increased recognition of the carer role. The organisation has also produced a number of publications that are closely linked to carer experiences. It also has a professionals' website for access to approaches to working with different carers.

www.carersuk.org

This is Carers UK, which is a national UK charity helping carers from all backgrounds by providing up-to-date information and advice about caring. This organisation also has a role in campaigning for better carers' rights and improving carers' lives. It is useful also for surveys on carers, reviewing different carer experiences and the latest research on carers as well as training days for both carers and professionals.

Chapter 8
Getting it right – the service user perspective

Sandra Walker and Dorothy Neal

NMC Standards for Pre-registration Nursing Education

This chapter will address the following competencies:

Domain 1: Professional values

2.1 **Mental health nurses** must practise in a way that addresses the potential power imbalances between professionals and people experiencing mental health problems, including situations when compulsory measures are used, by helping people exercise their rights, upholding safeguards and ensuring minimal restrictions on their lives. They must have an in depth understanding of mental health legislation and how it relates to care and treatment of people with mental health problems.

4. All nurses must work in partnership with service users, carers, groups, communities and organisations. They must manage risk, and promote health and wellbeing while aiming to empower choices that promote self-care and safety.

4.1 **Mental health nurses** must work with people in a way that values, respects and explores the meaning of their individual lived experiences of mental health problems, to provide person-centred and recovery-focused practice.

Domain 2: Communication and interpersonal skills

1. All nurses must build partnerships and therapeutic relationships through safe, effective and non-discriminatory communication. They must take account of individual differences, capabilities and needs.

1.1 **Mental Health Nurses** must use skills of relationship-building and communication to engage with and support people distressed by hearing voices, experiencing distressing thoughts or experiencing other perceptual problems.

2. All nurses must use a range of communication skills and technologies to support person-centred care and enhance quality and safety. They must ensure people receive all the information they need in a language and manner that allows them to make informed choices and share decision making. They must recognise when language interpretation or other communication support is needed and know how to obtain it.

Domain 3: Nursing practice and decision-making

8. All nurses must provide educational support, facilitation skills and therapeutic nursing interventions to optimise health and wellbeing. They must promote self-care and

continued . . .

management whenever possible, helping people to make choices about their healthcare needs, involving families and carers where appropriate, to maximise their ability to care for themselves.

8.1 **Mental health nurses** must practise in a way that promotes the self-determination and expertise of people with mental health problems, using a range of approaches and tools that aid wellness and recovery and enable self-care and self-management.

NMC Essential Skills Clusters

Cluster: Care, compassion and communication

1. As partners in the care process, people can trust a newly registered graduate nurse to provide collaborative care based on the highest standards, knowledge and competence.

By entry to the register:

12. Recognises and acts to overcome barriers in developing effective relationships with service users and carers.

2. People can trust the newly registered graduate nurse to engage in person centred care empowering people to make choices about how their needs are met when they are unable to meet them for themselves.

By entry to the register:

8. Is sensitive and empowers people to meet their own needs and make choices and considers with the person and their carer(s) their capability to care.

3. People can trust the newly registered graduate nurse to respect them as individuals and strive to help them to preserve their dignity at all times.

By entry to the register:

4. Acts professionally to ensure that personal judgements, prejudices, values, attitudes and beliefs do not compromise care.

Chapter aims

By the end of this chapter you should be able to:

- clearly understand how clinicians' behaviour has an impact on care delivery;
- consider ethical issues arising from a given clinical situation;
- reflect on your own values and judgements in interacting with service users in day-to-day care;
- have an increased understanding of the importance of validation and maintaining dignity in clinical care.

Introduction

The literature is littered with reviews, discussions and other evidence suggesting that in healthcare we do not always manage to engage and communicate in the best way (Francis, 2013). This chapter is slightly unusual in format in that it features one case study, comprising an interview carried out with a service user, Dorothy, following several years of care in a variety of clinical settings. Into this interview are interspersed activities, reflections and alternative case studies to help you to think more broadly around the issues raised within the interview itself.

A first encounter with mental health services

Q. Dorothy, could you give us a brief background of your MH history and the sort of services you have been involved with?

The first breakdown I had was when my step-dad died; it was awful, he took a long time to die and the hospital really weren't sympathetic; for my first death in the family it was very traumatic and I just fell to pieces, fell apart. I couldn't do anything, my husband took me to the GP; the first thing he said to me was 'How was your mother?' I thought, what! What are we talking about? I'm not here for my mother, I'm here for me. I was saying 'I don't think I'm going to be able to live'; I was completely destroyed and then he was grumpy because my time had run out so he just tutted and wrote a letter in silence then gave the letter to my husband and told him to take me to the local mental health hospital the next morning. That hospital was a scary place at that time; he hadn't explained anything to me and I didn't know whether to pack a bag or anything, I didn't know anything about it. It was really scary; he should have explained that I was going to see some team and that they would talk it over with me. So the next morning I went and saw some team, not sure who they were, but they were quite reassuring. I don't know how I got through that really, just antidepressants; the team were telling me I didn't have to go into hospital as I wasn't poorly enough. They told my husband he could leave me on my own and I didn't want to be left alone, it was terrifying the feelings I was going through. Looking back I think what needed to be done was I needed to be told what bereavement felt like – later I picked up a book which opened with 'No-one told me bereavement felt so much like fear.' That was so clear; if someone had sat me down and said 'You've just lost your dad, this is normal' and my mum kept saying 'You're going to end up in the mental hospital, stop crying, stop crying.' If someone, e.g. that GP, had just said to me this is what it feels like, it's OK to cry, to wail, to throw yourself on the floor like they do in other countries, I might have been OK really.

So the years ticked on; I was still on antidepressants, then I came off them to try and get pregnant. I got pregnant and had my son and then again I just fell apart. I couldn't sleep, I was so anxious. I was referred to the crisis team who kept telling me that there was nothing wrong and I could take care of my baby but that made it worse as I knew that there was something wrong. I was climbing the walls with anxiety about everything, about how to make his bottles, about everything. I just couldn't cope. With depression, it slows you down quite a lot, and being slowed down to that state and trying to take care of a newborn, it was hell, it really was, and the crisis team were supposed to be helping me and they just kept saying, 'There's nothing wrong with you, you're OK.' This went on for two weeks where I was just falling to bits. I didn't know what I was doing; finally, I made a call at 4 o'clock in the morning and said, 'I just cannot do it, I need to go into hospital' and this bloke said 'Do you know what, it's the time now, I think you're right' and it was such a breath of fresh air. They would talk about hospital, they're saying 'Oh you'll get institutionalised, you need to stay in the community', but this guy's attitude was 'You know, I think you've suffered enough, you need to go into hospital now.'

So I went to a mother and baby unit; I was terrified out of my wits, I was unable to chew my dinner, I just stood in a corner with my son; it wasn't explained to me that there would be other very unwell mothers in there with other illnesses. All I could see in there were mothers without babies; I thought they'd been taken away. So I just stood there and held him close, and eventually they came in and prised him out of my hand and then admitted me. I wasn't really taking everything in. Well, I was, it was sort of normal in my head. I wasn't psychotic, but I was slow on the outside and must have looked like a zombie, there were no facial movements. On the inside I was still there and that's one thing I wanted to get across that on the outside if we look like zombies, sometimes we're not there but mostly we are. I needed to have someone sit down and explain to me exactly what was going to happen, but they didn't do it, they just looked at me and it's as if they thought 'There's no point, she's not taking anything in', but I was taking everything in.

That first night I had a lovely Chinese nurse who managed to prise my son out of my hands, gave me a hot chocolate, then tucked me in bed and put the TV on for me, and it was so reassuring that: yes, I was a mother and I needed to take care of my child but I was also poorly and needed to be taken care of too. With the crisis team it was very much focused on 'You've got to take care of your baby' and I kept thinking 'But I'm ill and there's no one here to take care of me!' So the next day I saw the psychiatrist; he was better than the GP and did explain things very carefully; he reassured me regarding institutionalisation and medication, and he talked to me like I was all there, which I was. Then at the very end he said, 'Of course, if this was in the olden days, your baby would have been taken away, you'd have been locked upstairs in an attic somewhere and probably have jumped out of a window and killed yourself!' I thought, oh you were doing so well, how is that helpful to tell me that story? So I'm a mad woman who should be disowned by her family?

It was a mixed bag in there; what they needed was consistency because you get the shifts. I am a new mum, I've got a newborn and you get one lot of staff come in saying you must feed on demand and I didn't want to do that. I was very strong in my own mind I didn't want to do that; then another lot would come in and say it's OK to have a routine, then the next lot would come in and say no, no. I didn't know if I was coming or going. I remember one time when he was crying and they're going 'Feed him, feed him' really forcefully; I'm saying 'He's not hungry, he's tired' and in the end he fell asleep in one of the nurse's arms and she was like, 'Oh sorry.' It was good that she did say sorry. I mean, you're never going to get it right all of the time, but when you know you've got it really wrong, then just to have someone say sorry makes you feel a lot better. After I was discharged from there I found the crisis team hard work. They'd come and knock on the door and shout where they were from on the doorstop, and I'd be like 'Shut up and get in.' I didn't want my neighbours knowing. So I'd be there with two big blokes looking at me and I'd try and explain how hard it is looking after a newborn, you know, and they didn't know what to say. I don't really know, to this day, what their purpose is; it didn't help me at all.

I was referred to a community mental health team, with a psychiatrist who was OK; I've heard stories but he was OK with me; he took my case over, looked at my drugs. He was alright, just very practical and not really emotional, ' You're doing well, I'll see you again in 3/12', that sort of thing. So I ticked on and then I had a manic episode which was hard to see as I went up quite slowly and I first saw someone at the local walk-in centre as I'd had a chest infection and hadn't been to the doctor's. I had this awful, awful cough and I was completely run down where I had been burning the candle at both ends where the mania was just mild but it was there. Then I coughed once in town and the pain was horrendous and a shop assistant said 'You've cracked a rib.' So I went to the drop-in centre and I just could not stop crying, I was out of my mind; unfortunately, she wasn't a great help, telling me to calm down and to go and see my GP. Obviously, I didn't go and see my GP, so then I went high; at this point it was probably psychosis and the crisis team came out. It's all a bit hazy really; you can't remember a lot when you're high. So the crisis team came out and I don't know what they were doing; they'd just give me my tablets and my husband was dealing a lot with them but me, I just took my tablets as I knew if I didn't I'd end up in hospital. I mean, they're pretty unshockable; at times I was very rude to them and I think that was probably good as in that role I imagine you need to be pretty unshockable at the things you see and the things you hear.

Activity 8.1 — *Critical thinking*

Think over the text above.

- What issues have been raised here that you would consider to be most important from an engagement perspective?

An outline answer is provided at the end of the chapter.

When things go badly wrong

Q. Is there anything you could add from these experiences that would be a good example of them getting it really wrong?

I had to have a medical on the Mother and Baby Unit and one particular nurse asked me to strip to my underwear, so I did as I was told and laid on the bed. Then, without warning, she just put her hand inside my bra and checked my breasts and that was horrible. You're so vulnerable, she didn't tell me why she was doing it, she just did it and to this day I don't know what she was looking for, whether it was a breast lump or what. Sometimes, when you get admitted to psychiatric hospital you leave your dignity at the door; that was just so wrong for her to do that and not say 'Now I'm just going to examine you' and explain why. Just explaining step by step almost as if you were explaining to a child would have been better. I think we'd rather be patronised and explained to than treated like that and just not knowing what's going on. I would have rather she'd just explained 'Now I'm going to do this and you're going to have to do this'; that would have been a lot better rather than thinking I'm a zombie and it doesn't matter, she's not going to feel anything.

I think one of the main things I found is staff trying to tell you you're OK and not listening to the fact that I know me and I'm not OK. I went there for anxiety and I was so anxious, I'd just come out of the Mother and Baby Unit and I was so anxious but I was too scared to let that anxiety show as I thought I'd be straight back in there, so I kept it all tight in and didn't let it show, and they were like 'Oh there's nothing wrong with you, you shouldn't really be here' and not looking or listening, not looking outside the box; not everyone shows anxiety in the same way. If they'd relaxed with me just a bit, I probably would have been able to show what I was really going through and I would have got the help, but because I was so frightened I didn't do that. They tried cognitive behaviour therapy and I asked, 'Well, it's not working with me, what happens with people it doesn't work on?' The nurse said it works for everyone. Later, another nurse told me that was rubbish. I mean, you feel like an outsider anyway when you're mentally ill, so to feel like an outsider among outsiders is not good.

Activity 8.2   *Critical thinking*

Imagine yourself in a similar position.

- What is the effect of being treated that way, when staff keep saying there's nothing wrong?

Please see the end of the chapter for Dorothy's answer.

Q. So how should the team have approached you, do you think? What would have worked for you?

I think if they'd sat down and said there are a lot of people here very anxious, you don't look very anxious at all. Can you tell me a bit what's going on for you. If they'd looked a little bit deeper I'd have probably fallen to bits on them, which would have been a good thing as they could have helped put me back together again. It was a group setting, though, it wasn't one to one. I was terrified so I think it's just about getting back to explaining. It's not like a physical illness, is it? I mean, you've got six people in the group with broken arms you can say, right, you'll have a lot of pain for about three weeks, then it's going to go off and we'll take your cast off. Mental health is not like that, so we need to look at everyone as an individual and if someone looks OK, remember they are there for a reason, I haven't just walked in off the street to join them; they needed to dig a bit deeper and find out what's going on.

Activity 8.3   *Team working*

Dorothy has raised the issue of a lack of continuity within teams; multiple team members might visit a service user with no guarantee that the same person will be seen twice in one episode of care.

- What issues does this raise and what steps can a team take to address this issue?

An outline answer is provided at the end of the chapter.

An example of good practice

Q. Is there a particular situation where someone really got it right?

It was my health visitor; there was this awful meeting in my home where there were about eight professionals including her; I was sat in the middle and my son was there. These professionals were sat in my home asking me questions like 'Would you ever hurt your child?' and there's me saying 'It's really hard to speak in front of all of you.' I was terrified that they were going to take my son from me and afterwards my lovely health visitor came up to me. I didn't even tell her how I felt; she knew, she could see. She said 'I'm really sorry, that was really wrong' and even though it wasn't her who set up the meeting and it wasn't her fault, she just came to me again and said she was really sorry. So here I felt validated and that my voice had been heard. When you're mentally ill people do kind of sweep in and you lose control; having some of that control given back to you just makes your confidence better.

There was another really good thing when in the Mother and Baby Unit where another lovely nurse said, 'Is there anything I can help you with?' and I said 'Can you please just give me someone that's been through this' and like the very next day there's a lady sat on my bed who'd been through it, you know, and told me her story and that she'd come out the other end. That was wonderful, that was really, really important for me.

Another team I was involved with was an Early Intervention Team; they were a breath of fresh air, they listened, they tried to help, if you requested something they would go and do it, and if they couldn't do it they would have tried to help and they explained. I requested information for my son about my illness and they tried to find something; there wasn't much but they didn't try and fob me off. They are very positive, recovery focused; there was lots going on, they had a will to help really. They go away and you can see that they have tried to do what you requested. I always felt validated with them; they were empathetic and proactive. I always felt I was being listened to and taken seriously.

Research summary

A qualitative study by Eriksen et al. (2012) explored the experience of 11 people using community mental health services. In a series of 19 interviews they endeavoured to discover a little more about what sense and meaning was made of the interactions the participants had with their mental health professionals.

Findings

- *Shared humanity* – Service users reported that it was important that the professionals valued them as human beings and that there was a sense of shared humanity. This was shown by allowing the service users to see that the professionals are also human and imperfect, by openness about themselves to a certain point and receptiveness to the ideas and beliefs of the services user. Being indifferent, not understanding, or setting goals and agendas that are not the service users' detracts from the sense of value and shared humanity.

- *Sense of self* – It was also important to service users for staff to understand that in the presence of mental ill-health people may no longer feel like themselves. They are struggling to come to terms with a new 'me' and may feel they have to adjust to new limitations, so there is also a sense of working out new standards for their lives. The importance of professionals understanding and valuing the service users' work in this area cannot be overestimated, as part of our perceived value as human beings comes from others' opinions and beliefs about us. Hence, by being interested in and appreciating the work that a person is doing in building a new life, we can support the process more effectively.

- *Control* – In situations where service users may lose control, there was a reported sense of loss of esteem due to power imbalance. Services users spoke of only sharing things they felt the professional could manage, thus often finding themselves lonely and isolated. In some cases where the reaction of professionals was too controlling, the service users just locked down and shared nothing, and therefore were hindered significantly in the recovery process. A certain amount of control and needing to be active in their own care was important in combating this issue for service users.

- *Trusting relationships* – When professionals do understand and validate the service user experience, this helps them to feel more 'human' and can help manage the fear and frustration that often go hand in hand with mental ill-health. Service users reported that good professionals built trusting relationships and there was no need for the service users to hide aspects of themselves as they know the professional will respect their perspective and take them seriously. As human beings, our own sense of value is tied up with that of the value others hold of us. A feeling of connectivity and fellowship with others is an essential part of our humanity.

Being recognised as human and being valued by others is essential to all. In order for service users to be seen as human, professionals need to show themselves as human by giving something of themselves and 'walking in their shoes'. The concept of reciprocity is important in a caring relationship; growth happens on both sides of an encounter between two equal people. Care is not passively received; the service user and professional interests need to receive equal emphasis to promote an environment for recovery. The goal-oriented nature of mental health services is often counter-productive in creating this environment, emphasising the needs of the service above the needs of the service users.

Activity 8.4   *Reflection*

Think back over your time in practice.

- Can you pinpoint times where the needs of the service were clearly being put before the needs of the patient?
- Can you identify ways in which you could have done things differently in order to make the needs of the patient the priority?

As this is based on your own reflection, no outline answer is provided.

Communication

Q. Have there been any times when you have been really difficult to communicate with?

There have been times, once with the depression. I was in a very depressed state. When you're like that you can't communicate at all; you are so beaten down by the depression you can't articulate, it won't come out and at times you need to be prompted to be heard as you can go unnoticed. There were times in day treatment where the anxiety I was feeling just wasn't coming out, I was so anxious. It is at times like that that the feelings you have need to be teased out very gently and very sensitively. When people have done that, like pulling a little thread, and you get so far and it all comes flooding out. First of all, just persevere with the questions; you might be there for half an hour with one-word answers until you feel safe enough to really let it all out, that's the effect of the depression.

With the psychosis, when you're high, you just can't communicate. At that point I need to be cared for by someone else. You say all kinds of things, can be rude and obnoxious and you think you're better than everyone else. When you are that high, though, you still need to be treated with dignity and respect because you can look back and see how you were treated. Patience is needed in both cases, plus maintaining dignity and respect is really important.

Advice to student nurses

Q. What principles should a student mental health nurse consider with regard to engagement and communication?

I guess a lot of it comes with experience. They need to be unshockable, there's nothing worse than telling someone you trust something and them recoiling. To explain what they are doing, when you're depressed to remember that we are still there, we are not zombies or absent, we still know what's going on. Saying sorry when you get it wrong, it is a sensitive area. If someone had a broken leg and you as a student tripped over it you would say sorry; it's the same principle, if you make a mistake say sorry.

Conclusion

Patient reports vary as to the experience they receive during a care episode, but Taylor et al. (2009) recommend that more research evaluating the impact of care, particularly the psychosocial assessment and service users' experiences of this, is required. McHale and Felton (2010) conclude that there are clear discrepancies in the views of practitioners and service users of what constitutes a positive and negative attitude towards perceptions of care that need to be addressed. Service users continue to be dissatisfied with services, while services often believe that the care being provided is good. Tate (2010a), in her article describing one experience in the Emergency Department (ED) after she had injured herself, states that she had become used to ED staff 'getting it wrong'. The fact that they had done a good job on that occasion would stay with her for a long time. Examples of how staff can get it wrong include being judgemental, treating patients as time wasters, making assumptions and inappropriately demanding to see wounds (Tate, 2010b). Pembroke (2009) cites responses of staff as being frequently hostile and angry, and states that being given choice over treatment and decision making is essential for patients.

Self-harm

The challenging nature of self-harm provides a useful back-drop for the consideration of the issues raised in this interview. Redley (2010) undertook a qualitative study of 26 clinicians who had contact with patients who had overdosed, to consider how they made sense of their patients' overdoses. He found that clinicians constructed a 'normal' model of self-harm for more socially deprived patients, which was seen to be understandable in light of the hardship they must endure, but that this did not apply to more well-off patients who were viewed as having less hardship. The staff studied viewed suicidal acts as ultimately mysterious and unknowable, and they tried to avoid engaging with 'why' the self-harm had taken place as opposed to any other strategy. This professional distance, Redley (2010) hypothesises, may be an essential requirement for the emotional and psychological safety of the clinician. He points out that this 'point of view' may silence the patient and this certainly raises the issue of staff interpretation having a potentially detrimental effect on the patient's view of the assessment itself. Maddock et al. (2010) discovered that depressive motives for self-harm were viewed more sympathetically by both nurses and doctors than perceived 'manipulative' motives in their study looking at suicidal and non-suicidal self-harm in patients with borderline personality disorder. Mackay and Barrowclough (2005), while exploring perceptions of ED staff towards people who self-harm, found that if staff felt that the patient's self-harm was triggered by a factor they felt was controllable in some way, for example substance misuse, they were more likely to be irritated and frustrated with the patient and less likely to be optimistic and helpful.

Chapter summary

Dealing with human beings in distress is a difficult and sensitive undertaking. It is easy to get it wrong. There are, however, certain points raised in this chapter that, if upheld during your practice, will help you to ensure that you do not stray far from the path of being a caring and effective practitioner. These echo *The Code* as laid out for you by the NMC (2008).

Treating people with respect, ensuring their dignity is upheld, having an open, honest interest in their position, keeping them at the heart of care delivery and ensuring they have an opportunity to direct the care they need will help to make sure you are providing excellent person-centred care.

Activities: brief outline answers

Activity 8.1: Critical thinking (page 133)

Look beyond the surface.

- Damage of invalidation – The GP undermined the importance of Dorothy's feelings by comparing them with her mother's at the time of bereavement. The crisis team kept telling her she was OK when she clearly did not feel OK.
- Respect for the person as a fellow human being – The patient has some intelligence and is an expert in his or her own state, even when suffering psychomotor retardation, as in depression in this case.
- Poor communication – Dorothy's anxiety was repeatedly raised just because the processes and changes in the care/team were not explained to her.
- Normalisation of feelings, e.g. bereavement.
- Importance of consistency of approach.

Activity 8.2: Critical thinking (page 134)

You are not listened to, your feelings aren't validated, which makes you feel worse. I mean, you've lost your confidence and it makes you lose your confidence even more. It makes you feel even more ill, people are saying you're alright and you're like, 'I'm not alright.' If people actually sat you down and said 'You're really poorly' and validated it, when that man did say that it was like 'At last, someone's listening to me!' and it is almost soothing, it gives you more anxiety when someone says 'You're fine, you're fine, there's nothing wrong', then you think maybe everyone feels like this and maybe I'm pathetic and just can't deal with it.

Activity 8.3: Team working (page 135)

Issues raised might include communications issues, poor care delivery due to lack of cohesion among staff regarding care plans, reduced possibility of creating a therapeutic alliance with the service user, increased anxiety for the service user having to meet new people, and the possibility of repeated assessment and having to explain multiple times her or his mental state.

One of the things teams could do in order to address these issues are to allocate a key working team wherever possible, ensuring that the same group of people go to see the service user, thus hopefully providing at least one familiar face at each visit. Careful time management and scheduling of visits can assist here. High documentation standards are also essential, to ensure that information is being shared within the whole team and every team member must commit to reading the notes and care plans on each person regularly to ensure they are up to date. Regular team meetings where cases are discussed are also essential so that cohesion and consistency of care are maximised.

Activity 8.5: Communication (page 138)

- Hear the patient – Listen and do not prejudge or think of the person as bad or badly behaved. Remember that something has happened to trigger the arousal and we need to discover what that is.
- Explain what the rules are and the reasons behind them – Ideally this should be done while the person is calm; however, once the person is aroused it can still be done in clear terms without using jargon or raising one's voice.
- 'Don't argue or confront' gained equal billing with 'give choices, empower' – Both were considered equally important in communicating with highly aroused people.
- NB: Forceful containment was also considered on the list in the document, but here we have not included it as there is not time to consider the wider ethical considerations of this subject. These are noted in the text of the document itself.

Further reading

Bowers, L, Brennan, G, Winship, G and Theodoridou, C (2009) *Talking With Acutely Psychotic People.* London: City University. Available online at www.iop.kcl.ac.uk/iopweb/blob/downloads/locator/l_436_Talking.pdf (accessed 14 June 2014).

This is a study that aimed to explore the techniques that professionals, working with people who are mentally ill, employ to enable good communication to occur despite the difficulties of the mental state of the individual.

Commission on Dignity in Care for Older People (2012) *Delivering Dignity.* Available online at www.nhsconfed.org/Documents/dignity.pdf (accessed 12 March 2013).

This is a document that, although primarily aimed at older persons' care, has many transferable issues for the care of any human being.

Reed, A (2011) *Nursing in Partnership with Patients and Carers*. Exeter: Learning Matters.

This is a useful guide to working partnerships with patients and carers that challenges us to see the person in the patient and promotes participation in care.

Reynolds, J, Muston, R, Heller, T, Leach, J, McCormick, M, Wallcraft, J and Walsh, M (eds) (2009) *Mental Health Still Matters*. Basingstoke: Palgrave Macmillan.

This is a collection of readings that challenge views about how to best understand and explain mental distress. Many chapters are written by service users and the whole book provides a challenge to traditional understandings of healthcare delivery.

Useful websites

www.invo.org.uk

Involve is a national advisory group that supports greater public involvement in NHS, public health and social care research.

www.mind.org.uk

Mind is a charity devoted to ensuring that anyone with a mental health problem has somewhere to turn for advice and support.

www.time-to-change.org.uk

This is a website that aims to end mental health discrimination. It contains a wealth of useful resources including short films and blogs where people who have experienced mental distress share their stories.

References

Akerjordet, K and Severinsson, E (2004) Emotional intelligence in mental health nurses talking about practice. *International Journal of Mental Health Nursing*, 13: 164–70.

American Psychiatric Association (APA) (2013) *Diagnostic and Statistical Manual for Mental Disorders, 5th Revision*. Washington: American Psychiatric Association.

Aseltine, RH and DeMartino, R (2004) An outcome evaluation of the SOS Suicide Prevention Program. *American Journal of Public Health*, 94(3): 446–51.

Aslan, M and Smith, M (2012) Promoting health and social inclusion, in Tee, S, Brown, J and Carpenter, D (eds) *Handbook of Mental Health Nursing*. London: Hodder Arnold.

Barber, P, Brown, R and Martin, D (2012) *Mental Health Law in England and Wales: A guide for mental health professionals* (2nd edition). London: Learning Matters.

Bear, MF, Connors, BW and Paradiso, MA (2007) *Neuroscience: Exploring the brain* (3rd edition). London: Lippincott Williams & Wilkins.

Beck, JS (1995) *Cognitive Therapy: Basics and beyond*. New York: Guilford.

Bennett-Levy, J (2006) Therapist skills: a cognitive model of their acquisition and refinement. *Behavioural and Cognitive Psychotherapy*, 37(1): 57–78.

Bennett-Levy, J, Turner, F, Beaty, T, Smith, M, Paterson, B and Farmer, S (2001) The value of self-practice of cognitive therapy techniques and self-reflection in the training of cognitive therapists. *Behavioural and Cognitive Psychotherapy*, 29: 203–20.

Bernard, JM and Goodyear, RK (2004) *Fundamentals of Clinical Supervision*. Boston, MA: Pearson Education.

Bhui, K, McCabe, R, Weich, S, Singh, S, Johnson, M and Szczpura, A (2013) THERACOM: A systematic review of the evidence base for interventions to improve therapeutic communications between black and minority ethnic populations and staff in specialist mental health services. *BioMedCentral: Systematic Reviews*, 2(1): Article No. 15.

Bowers, L, Brennan, G, Winship, G and Theodoridou, C (2009) *Talking With Acutely Psychotic People: Communication skills for nurses and others spending time with people who are very mentally ill*. London: City University. Available online at www.iop.kcl.ac.uk/iopweb/blob/downloads/locator/l_436_Talking.pdf (accessed 14 June 2014).

Bowers, L, Brennan, G, Winship, G and Theodoridou, C (2010) How expert nurses communicate with acutely psychotic patients. *Mental Health Practice*, 13(7): 24–6.

Brown, J (2012) The therapeutic use of self, in Tee, S, Brown, J and Carpenter, D (eds) *Handbook of Mental Health Nursing*. London: Hodder Arnold.

Brown, P, Calnan, M, Scriver, A and Szmukler, G (2009) Trust in mental health services: a neglected concept. *Journal of Mental Health*, October 18(5): 449–58.

Buckner, L and Yeandle, S (2011) *Valuing Carers 2011: Calculating the value of carers' support*. London: Carers UK.

Cahill, J, Barkham, M, Hardy, G, Gilbody, S, Richards, D, Bower, P, Audin, K and Connell, J (2008) A review and critical appraisal of measures of therapist–patient interactions in mental health settings. *Health Technology Assessment*, 12(24).

Campinha-Bacote, J (2002) The process of cultural competence in the delivery of healthcare services: a model of care. *Journal of Transcultural Nursing*, 13(3): 181–4.

Carers Trust (2012) *What Is a Carer?* Available online at www.carers.org/what-carer (accessed 4 August 2012).

Castledine, G (2010) Creative nursing: art or science? *British Journal of Nursing*, 19(14): 937.

Chadwick, P (2006) *Person-based Cognitive Therapy for Distressing Psychosis.* Chichester: John Wiley & Sons.

Commissioning Board, Chief Nursing Officer and Department of Health Chief Nursing Adviser (2012) *Compassion in Practice.* Available online at www.commissioningboard.nhs.uk (accessed 13 October 2013).

Cross, WM and Bloomer, MJ (2010) Extending boundaries: clinical communication with culturally and linguistically diverse mental health clients and carers. *International Journal of Mental Health Nursing*, 19(4): 268–77.

Cummings, J. (2012) *Compassion in Practice: Nursing, midwifery and care staff – our vision and strategy.* London: NHS Commissioning Board.

De Bellis, A, Bradley, SL, Wotherspoon, A, Walter, B, Guerin, P, Cecchin, M and Paterson, J (2009) *Come Into My World: How to interact with a person who has dementia: An educational resource for undergraduate healthcare students on person-centred care.* Adelaide: Flinders University. Available online at http://nursing.flinders.edu.au/comeintomyworld (accessed 27 October 2013).

Deegan, PE (1988) Recovery: the lived experience of rehabilitation. *Psychosocial Rehabilitation Journal*, 11(4): 11–19.

Department of Health (DH) (2005a) *NIMHE Guiding Statement on Recovery.* London: DH.

Department of Health (DH) (2005b) *Delivering Race Equality in Mental Health Care: An action plan for reform inside and outside services and the government's response to the independent inquiry into the death of David Bennett.* London: HMSO.

Department of Health (DH) (2007) *Capabilities for Inclusive Practice.* London: DH.

Department of Health (DH) (2008a) *High Quality Care for All.* London: DH.

Department of Health (DH) (2008b) *Carers at the Heart of the 21st Century: Families and communities.* London: HMSO.

Department of Health (DH) (2012) *Caring for Our Future: Reforming care and support.* London: HMSO.

Diederen, KMJ, Daalman, K, De Weijer, AD, Neggers, SFW, Van Gastel, W, Dirk Blom, J, Kahnl, RS and Sommer, IEC (2011) Auditory hallucinations elicit similar brain activations in psychotic and nonpsychotic individuals. *Schizophrenia Bulletin*, 38(5): 1074–82.

Dietrich, S, Wittenburg, L, Arensman, E, Värnik, A and Hegerl, U (2009) Suicide and self-harm, in Gask, L, Lester, H, Kendrick, T and Peveler, R (eds) *Primary Care Mental Health.* London: Royal College of Psychiatrists, pp125–45.

Driscoll, J (1994) Reflective practice for practise. *Senior Nurse*, 13: 47–50.

Egan, G (2010) *The Skilled Helper: A problem-management and opportunity-development approach to helping* (10th edition). Belmont, CA: Brooks/Cole.

Egan, G (2013) *The Skilled Helper* (10th edition). Belmont, CA: Brooks Cole.

Eriksen, KA, Sundfor, B, Karlsson, B, Raholm, MB and Arman, M (2012) Recognition as a valued human being: perspectives of mental health service users. *Nursing Ethics*, 19(3): 357–68.

Fernando, S (2010) *Mental Health, Race and Culture* (3rd edition). Basingstoke: Palgrave Macmillan.

Francis, R (Chair) (2013) *Report of the Mid Staffordshire NHS Foundation Trust Public Enquiry.* London: The Stationery Office.

Freshwater, D and Stickley, T (2004) The heart of the art: emotional intelligence in nurse education. *Nurse Inquiry*, 11(2): 91–8.

Gerrish, K, Husband, C and Mackenzie, J (1996) *Nursing for a Multi-ethnic Society.* Buckingham: Open University Press.

Gibbs, G (1988) *Learning by Doing: A guide to teaching and learning methods.* Oxford: Oxford Polytechnic.

Hatfield, A (1994) The family's role in caregiving and service delivery, in Lefley, H and Wasom, M (eds) *Helping Families Cope with Mental Illness.* Newark, NJ: Harwood Academic Publishers.

Heron, J (2001) *Helping the Client* (5th edition). London: Sage.

Hope, R (2004) *The Ten Essential Shared Capabilities: A framework for the whole of the mental health workforce.* London: Department of Health.

Horvath, AO and Greenberg, LS (eds) (1994) *The Working Alliance: Theory, research, and practice.* New York: Wiley.

Horvath, AO and Luborsky, L (1993) The role of the therapeutic alliance in psychotherapy. *Journal of Consulting and Clinical Psychology*, 61(4): 561–73.

Johns, C (1995) The value of reflective practice for nursing. *Journal of Clinical Nursing*, 4: 23–30.

Kitwood, T (1997) *Dementia Reconsidered: The person comes first.* Buckingham: Open University Press.

Kolb, D (1984) *Experimental Learning.* Englewood Cliffs, NJ: Prentice Hall.

Lipson, JG (1999) Cross-cultural nursing: the cultural perspective. *Journal of Transcultural Nursing*, 10(1): 6.

Luborsky, L, Rosenthal, R, Diguer, L, Andrusyna, TP, Berman, JS, Levitt, JT, Seligman, DA and Krause, ED (2002) The Dodo bird verdict is alive and well – mostly. *Clinical Psychology: Science and Practice*, 9(1): 2–12.

Mackay, N and Barrowclough, C (2005) A&E staff's perception of DSH: attributions, emotions and willingness to help. *British Journal of Clinical Psychology*, 44: 255–67.

Maddock, GR, Carter, GL, Murrell, ER, Lewin, TJ and Conrad, AM (2010) Distinguishing suicidal from non-suicidal deliberate self-harm events in women with borderline personality disorder. *Australian & New Zealand Journal of Psychiatry*, 44: 574–82.

Marieb, EN and Hoehn, K (2010) *Human Anatomy & Physiology* (8th edition). London: Benjamin Cummings.

McHale, J and Felton, A (2010) Self-harm: what's the problem? A literature review of the factors affecting attitudes towards self-harm. *Journal of Psychiatric & Mental Health Nursing*, 17: 732–40.

Mead, N and Bower, P (2002) Patient-centred consultations and outcomes in primary care: a review of the literature. *Patient Education and Counselling*, 48(1): 51–61.

Mental Health Foundation (2014) *Recovery.* Available online at www.mentalhealth.org.uk/help-information/mental-health-a-z/R/recovery (accessed 4 March 2014).

Middlewick, Y (2013) Engaging the person, in Walker, S, Carpenter, D and Middlewick, Y (eds) *Assessment and Decision Making in Mental Health Nursing.* London: Sage/Learning Matters.

Middlewick, Y and Carpenter, D (2013) Outcomes of assessment, in Walker, S, Carpenter, D and Middlewick, Y (eds) *Assessment and Decision Making in Mental Health Nursing.* London: Sage/Learning Matters.

Milne, D (2009) *Evidence-based Clinical Supervision: Principles and practice.* Chichester: BPS Blackwell.

Mind (2011) *Listening to Experience*. London: Mind. Available online at www.mind.org.uk/campaigns_and_issues/report_and_resources/6051_listening_to_experience (accessed 7 October 2013).

Mind (2013) *Nearest Relatives under the Mental Health Act*. London: Mind. Available online at www.mind.org.uk/mental_health_a-z/8064_nearest_relatives_under_the_mental_health_act (accessed 27 January 2013).

Morgan, C, Burns, T, Fitzpatrick, R, Pinfold, V and Priebe, S (2007) Social exclusion and mental health: conceptual and methodological review. *British Journal of Psychiatry*, 191: 477–83.

Murphy, R and Wales, P (2013) *Mental Health Law in Nursing*. London: Sage/Learning Matters.

Myles, P and Rushforth, D (2007) *A Complete Guide to Primary Care Mental Health*. London: Robinson.

National Black Carers and Carers Workers Network (NBCCWN) (2008) *Beyond We Care Too: Putting black carers in the picture*. London: Afiya Trust.

National Collaborating Centre for Mental Health (2012) *Service User Experience in Adult Mental Health* (CG 136). Leicester and London: British Psychological Society and Royal College of Psychiatrists. Published online in December 2011 at www.nice.org.uk/nicemedia/live/13629/57542/57542.pdf (accessed June 2013).

National Institute for Health and Clinical [now Care] Excellence (NICE) (2005) *Violence: The short term management of disturbed/violent behaviour in in-patient psychiatric settings and emergence departments* (CG 25). London: NICE.

Norman, I (2009) The art and science of mental health nursing: reconciliation of two traditions in the cause of public health. *International Journal of Nursing Studies*, 46: 1537–40.

Norman, IJ and Ryrie, I (2013) *The Art and Science of Mental Health Nursing: Principles and practice* (3rd edition). Maidenhead: Open University Press.

Nursing and Midwifery Council (NMC) (2008) *The Code: Standards of conduct, performance and ethics for nurses and midwives*. London: NMC. Available online at www.nmc-uk.org/Documents/Standards/The-code-A4-20100406.pdf (accessed 14 June 2013).

Nursing and Midwifery Council (NMC) (2010a) *Standards for Pre-registration Nursing Education*. London: NMC. Available online at http://standards.nmc-uk.org/Pages/Welcome.aspx (accessed 2 December 2013).

Nursing and Midwifery Council (NMC) (2010b) *Essential Skills Clusters and Guidance for Their Use* (Guidance G7.1.5b). Available online at www.standards.nmc-uk.org/Documents/Annexe3_%20ESCs_16092010.pdf (accessed 12 June 2013).

O'Brien, A, Famy, R and Singh, S (2009) Disengagement from mental health services: a literature review. *Social Psychiatry and Psychiatric Epidemiology*, 44: 558–68.

O'Carroll, M and Park, A (2007) *Essential Mental Health Skills*. Philadelphia, PA: Mosby Elsevier.

Padesky, CA and Greenberger, D (1996) *Mind Over Mood*. New York: Guilford Press.

Pearce, R (2006) Communicating and relating, in Trenoweth, S, Docherty, T and Price, I (eds) *Nursing and Mental Health Care: An introduction for all fields of practice*. Exeter: Learning Matters.

Pembroke, L (2009) Them and us? How education and training can improve relationships between psychiatrists and service users. *Open Mind*, 157: 14.

Peplau, HE (1952) *Interpersonal Relations in Nursing*. New York: GP Putnam & Sons.

Priebe, S, Watts, J, Chase, M and Matanov, A (2005) Processes of disengagement and engagement in assertive outreach patients: qualitative study. *The British Journal of Psychiatry*, 187: 438–43.

Prochaska, JO and DiClemente, CC (1983) Stages and processes of self-change of smoking: toward an integrative model of change. *Journal of Consulting and Clinical Psychology*, 5 (3): 390–5.

Redley, M (2010) The clinical assessment of patients admitted to hospital following an episode of self-harm: a qualitative study. *Sociology of Health and Illness*, 32(3): 1–16.

Repper, J (2012) Recovery: a journey of discovery, in Tee, S, Brown, J and Carpenter, D (eds) *Handbook of Mental Health Nursing*. London: Hodder Arnold.

Richards, D and Whyte, R (2011) *Reach Out: National programme student materials to support the delivery of training for psychological wellbeing practitioners delivering low intensity interventions* (3rd edition). London: Rethink.

Rogers, C (1957) The necessary and sufficient conditions of therapeutic personality change. *Journal of Consulting Psychology*, 21(2): 95–103.

Rogers, C (1959) A theory of therapy, personality and interpersonal relationships as developed in the client-centered framework, in Koch, S (ed.) *Psychology: A study of a science. Vol. 3: Formulations of the person and the social context*. New York: McGraw Hill.

Rogers C (1961) *On Becoming a Person*. Boston, MA: Houghton Mifflin.

Roth, A and Pilling, S (2007) *The Competences Required to Deliver Effective Cognitive and Behavioural Therapy for People with Depression and with Anxiety Disorders*. London: Department of Health. Available online at www.ucl.ac.uk/clinical-psychology/CORE/CBT_Competences/CBT_Competence_List.pdf (accessed 12 June 2013).

Royal College of Psychiatrists (RCPsych) (2009) *Mental Health and Social Inclusion: Making psychiatry and mental health services fit for the 21st century*. London: RCPsych. Available online at www.rcpsych.ac.uk/pdf/social%20inclusion%20position%20statement09.pdf (accessed 13 June 2013).

Shattell, MM, Starr, SS and Thomas, SP (2007) Take my hand, help me out: mental health service recipients' experiences of the therapeutic relationship. *International Journal of Mental Health Nursing*, 16: 274–84.

Shepherd, G, Boardman, J and Slade, M (2008) *Making Recovery a Reality*. London: Sainsbury's Centre for Mental Health (SCMH).

Simon, RI and Hales, RE (eds) (2012) *American Psychiatric Publishing Textbook of Suicide Assessment and Management*. Arlington, VA: APA.

Social Care Institute for Excellence (SCIE) (2005) *SCIE Research Briefing 11: The health and well-being of young carers*. London, SCIE.

Social Exclusion Unit (2004) *Mental Health and Social Exclusion: Social Exclusion Unit report*. London: Office of the Deputy Prime Minister. Available online at www.socialfirmsuk.co.uk/resources/library/mental-health-and-social-exclusion-social-exclusion-unit-report (accessed 14 June 2013).

Spector, RE (2004) *Cultural Diversity in Health and Illness* (6th edition). Englewood Cliffs, NJ: Pearson-Prentice Hall.

Tate, A (2010a) Getting it right: caring for people who self-harm. *Emergency Nurse*, 18(6): 32–3.

Tate, A (2010b) A private matter. *Emergency Nurse*, 18(4): 11.

Taylor, TL, Hawton, K, Fortune, S and Kapur, N (2009) Attitudes towards clinical services among people who self-harm: systematic review. *British Journal of Psychiatry*, 194: 104–10.

Van Dusseldorp, LRLC, Van Meijel, BKG and Derksen, JJL (2010) Emotional intelligence in mental health nurses. *Journal of Clinical Nursing*, 20: 555–62.

Van Lutterveld, R, Diederen, KMJ, Koops, S, Begemann, MJH and Sommer, IEC (2013) The influence of stimulus detection on activation patterns during auditory hallucinations. *Schizophrenia Research*, 145: 27–32.

Vercammen, A, Knegtering, H, Bruggeman, R and Aleman, A (2011) Subjective loudness and reality of auditory verbal hallucinations and activation of the inner speech processing network. *Schizophrenia Bulletin*, 37(5): 1009–16.

Walker, S, Carpenter, D and Middlewick, Y (2013) *Assessment and Decision Making in Mental Health Nursing.* London: Sage/Learning Matters.

Westbrook, D, Kennerley, H and Kirk, J (2011) *An Introduction to Cognitive Behaviour Therapy* (2nd edition). London: Sage.

Williams, A (2013) *The Listening Organisation*. Cardiff: 1000 Lives Plus.

Worden, JW (2009) *Grief Counselling and Grief Therapy: A handbook for the mental health practitioner* (4th edition). Oxford: Routledge.

Index